The Previous Essays of a Former Paranoid Schizophrenic

"Highrise Two"

103 Stories

I0103278

Milo Seamus Miles

chipmunkapublishing
the mental health publisher

Milo Seamus Miles

All rights reserved, no part of this publication may be reproduced by any means, electronic, mechanical photocopying, documentary, film or in any other format without prior written permission of the publisher.

Published by
Chipmunkapublishing
PO Box 6872
Brentwood
Essex CM13 1ZT
United Kingdom

http://www.chipmunkapublishing.com

Copyright © Milo S. Miles 2009

Chipmunkapublishing gratefully acknowledge the support of Arts Council England.

THE PREVIOUS ESSAYS OF A FORMER PARANOID SCHIZOPHRENIC

In Memoriam

Pauline Nolan

1947-1998

Milo Seamus Miles

THE PREVIOUS ESSAYS OF A FORMER PARANOID SCHIZOPHRENIC

1. Dung

At Zaire National Zoo Ossie Stretch the ostrich keeper was busy on a personal matter. "What's the matter?" you may ask. "No matter," he'd reply, "It doesn't matter". But it did matter, and what Ossie wanted no-one to know was that he was stealing elephant droppings, putting them in a trunk, and sending them on ahead of the elephant to the studio of a very famous artist in England, to be displayed on canvas with the artist's work and exhibited in art galleries throughout that country and beyond.

Of course Ossie, if it was discovered it was he who was providing the elephant faeces, would be in the shit for not sharing his remuneration with the zoo authorities. Why put Ossie at risk when perfectly formed elliedung was available at zoos throughout the U.K.? It came out that the consistency of the product is different in Zaire, due to the elephant having the more 'natural' diet available in Africa. This made it particularly appealing for the artist's palate. "It's a question of quality, as connoisseurs of this artist material will know," quipped the painter, "You have to pay through the nose to get a trunkful of elephant's excrement".

2. Some Clergy

Bishop Basher was a matey of the laity. He also liked to think he had friends in sky places, especially after two or three spirits in the evening prior to taking his dog 'Collar' for a walk. On one such walk he bumped into the Rev. Mick McVicar, who had just met Father Seamus O'Reilly at a ball in the Parish Hall. Mick had said, "I'm Reverend McVicar. What's your name?" Seamus had replied "O'Reilly". At this Mick had said "Oh really!", Seamus responded "No, O'Reilly". They had laughed over this quip, and had great fun telling the Bishop of it.

The three of them had started to discuss the divisions between the Anglican and Roman Catholic churches, which hadn't been helped by the recent scandal of a local priest running off with the vicar's wife. She had apparently been defrocked and the priest was unfrocked.
The curious curate asked the Right Reverend if the wronged reverend had forgiven the marriage vows transgressors. The Bishop replied that the spurned prelate often prayed for their and our souls.

3. A Sovereign

Windsor Castle lived with Sybil Lyst. She supported him and their son Buckingham in style, while the extended family existed on generous state handouts. The family enjoyed public popularity a lot of the time, due to the personal touch of the official matriarch. Sybil was dynamic, there could be no doubting of that, for she was often seen in near and far-flung places, making the public appearances that were the bread and butter of her perceived role, that is that of an important personage.

Unfortunately for her she had no personal power, only a few rights, for example the right to be consulted, the right to encourage, and the right to warn the Prime Minister, who ultimately decided what was to be proposed to Parliament and passed with his party's majority. Her influence, though, should not be underestimated, as she evoked the respect due to someone who had knowledge of the personal habits of several British Prime Ministers, dozens of world figures, not to say statesmen, and hundreds of opportunistic, scheming, grasping and greedy persons who became prominent from time to time, as well as the humble people who were rewarded by 'her' gift, the honours connected with the British Empire, whatever that is, in return for their service; also lots that weren't.

The fact that no British Prime Minister has tried to get Sybil replaced as Head of State must prove that she is thought to be of use.

4. Neighbours

Ben and Den Zen were religious men. Mick, Vick and Nick Bick were Catholic. Dan, Ann and Fran Chan were Anglican. Sid, Cyd and their kids were Yiddish. Yet despite the diversity of their spiritual beliefs, they stuck together in adversity, with the desired outcome coming about, I shout. They had raised funds for charity part-time by selling braised food for the multitude of neighbours in the neighbourhood, hoods excluded. They were united in opposing the disease cancer, that death enhancer, as so much can be done these days to combat it, hopefully even more given research, in the future with the finance.

Dan and Den got together again at the New Forest Gumph Golf Club, playing around so much that they couldn't concentrate on their golf. The sound of the skylarking had the dogs barking angrily in the vicinity in unison and unity. One cannot annoy canines with impunity as if one had diplomatic immunity from their reactions, for they might bite.

While Dan and Den were busy with the golf clubs at the golf club, Den's big brother Ben was counting to ten to stop his affection for Dan's wife Ann becoming obvious to Ann and Fran, their daughter. Ben was a gardener, doing the Chans' garden, mostly lawn, but some topiary since before Fran was born, including this day. Ann and Cyd had invited Ben to take a break and join them for a cup of tea, to discuss plans to fund raise for their favourite, already mentioned, charity. Although only a humble artisan, Ben was well motivated in this, for the first girl he had kissed (she was a Miss Trish Fish and a dish) had succumbed to a carcinoma, and he had dedicated his deeds accordingly in her memory. Besides, he liked and would have loved his neighbours given the chance, religious scruples apart, and now Mick and Vick Bick had joined them, bringing some biscuits. "Mickey would you like a bicky?" said Ann. "How about you others?" It was proposed they have a fun day on a future Sunday at the nearby day school, which they used as a rule as it was cool in the shade in summer. Possible viable attractions were listed, while Fran persisted in plying refreshments on her Mum's guests at her behest as her contribution to proceedings.

After discussion about Prussian percussion and Russian recession when planning for the fun day had ceased, Ben made his excuses and went back to weeding out-of-place flowers. Nick came home from schooling with Cyd's kids, drooling over Vicky's bickys, when transport brought Den and Dan home from their sport. At this meeting the greeting was great, as if it were an important date. The fun day and a fête would have to wait; there was a need for friendship to satiate.

What about Sid, you say? He had hidden in the hay on the farm that he ran, to check on the labouring types. He found one a little lazy, so much so that if he'd been in the army it would have cost him his stripes. Lucky for him Sid fell asleep, and he was warned by his snoring. So although he found his work boring, as he needed the wages for whoring he'd better get on with what he found abhorring.

So Sid was in the land of nod while his God-fearing friends frolicked in a frenzy. No, not really; they just chuckled in the deep full-throated way individuals satisfied with their lot used to show their appreciation of others.

5. A Marriage

"Hilary Beverley Lesley Vivian Ponsonby, I hereby declare you married to Molly Polly Dolly Jolly. May you have a happy life together". These were the words ringing in the ears of the couple as the cheers of the witnesses began.

With a break for a short time of intimate privacy together, Hilary and Molly then proceeded to the lavish reception, for no expense had been spared. The photographers were here at Amsterdam Register Office, during the ceremony and afterwards on the steps. Hundreds of pictures were taken to accompany the thousands of words that journalists would write about this beautiful couple's coupling together legally. The gutter press' gossip columnists were well represented.

Hilary, in a kilt, and Molly, in a pink silk creation, welcomed the attention, as payment for coverage had been made and paid for, and more, the entire day.

The partners hobnobbed with minor celebrities, as well as obscure, exotically dressed, not to say erotically dressed, representatives of various parties involved in their busy social life back in London and the Home Counties, before flying off for two weeks of sexual gratification and sight-seeing around Cairo, Egypt.

THE PREVIOUS ESSAYS OF A FORMER PARANOID SCHIZOPHRENIC

They were just like any other honeymooners in Luxor, by the Pyramids and the Sphinx. Molly actually told Hilary "I think the Sphinx stinks". To which Hilary replied "No dear, we are downwind of the rear of that camel".

The only fly in the ointment was that their marriage was not recognised by the Egyptian authorities, despite the fact that a change in the law in Holland had allowed them to be the first two females to marry each other.

6. All Wright, Brothers!

Jumping beans, jumping queues, is it any wonder I've got the blues? In the critics' reviews I receive the worst news. They say I cannot write; this is wrong, I have every right to pursue life, liberty, and happiness, and bless every being I encounter, even the third kind with the product of my pen I reiterate, say again, I have talent. I have latent abilities that would stagger you to such an extent you'd fall over if you conceived their size.

It would be such a surprise, it would really open your eyes from being blind, you would have a superhero's sight, x-ray and all that. But I'm such a cool cat, jumping Jehosaphat, so laid back it stops me in my tracks from announcing to all that I have genius, like that character Oscar Wilde, only straight. It's not too late to be a future great, make masterpieces with imagination and ink. You try it too, we'll be fab us two, we have to.

It's our duty to make every life a beauty, using body, mind, soul; perfection is our goal. Start right here, forget your fear, cheer, go for it, be brave, if you are a Brave be a courageous Brave. Wherever you're from, return or stay with honour, don't stray from righteousness, be a goner. You know what's wrong, avoid it, sing your own song, be devoid of bad, therefore happy not sad. What little else I can say pales into insignificance, so it's time to call it a day, time to choreograph a new dance. The Lord is the tunesmith, the lyrics are mine.

THE PREVIOUS ESSAYS OF A FORMER PARANOID SCHIZOPHRENIC

7. The Circus

Moustachioed Mustapha the Magnificent was known for his munificence in circuses throughout countries of the civilised continent. His regard for Rosie, the bareback rider, was legendary. He had really fallen.

But he had a rival, Ronald the ringmaster, whose need for power was freakish. While Mustapha tamed the tigers, Ron tried to tame Rosie recklessly.

Passing the big top at twenty-two ticks past twelve our Must found Rosie had given Ron his come-comeuppance. Miserly with his money, he had flourished for her flowers that had only cost him tuppence. She had hurled them at his head and stomped to her caravan for bed, 'twas then she met Mustapha who said, "I do love you dearly, ducky. I like it when you get clucky. Do let's get wed next Wednesday week, in time for tea. I'll get a special licence and you may make a he-man out of me."

Our hero and his mate made that marriage date and tied the knot in the big top, while mean Ronald retired to Reigate to run a ruddy flea-circus ruinously.

8. Not All There

Let them eat bread till they're dead, if they eat cake they may awake, realise their plight. We live in the sun, they live in the night. Pop music is the opium of the masses; the religious pay their taxes. We live charmed lives, while they have a semblance, a guise. They deserve their misery; they are not aware, not really sane. I blame their upbringing.

Singing alleviates their suffering. Education encourages equality, but not at the expense of integrity. Pursuing solving personal problems is a premier prerequisite of passing time. No matter what situation in life you're at, the human condition is common. May one find salvation in the correction of mistakes and inherited difficulties.

9. Awareness

Generals genuflecting before gentlewomen
manners maketh the man
in this citizen's civilisation
this people's paradise
human beings beg to be excused
they say "Pardon me, fiddle-de-dee
I do beg your pardon".
We feign to forgive bad form.
Civility costs nothing, the higher
the class the more is expected.
Crassness just won't do.
So what's it to you
when rude ruffians behave badly?
I suppose it's usually upsetting
but even if you are brutish, brutalised
and insensitive, not knowing any etiquette
at all, you may still be offended
by the attitude of the transgressor.
One needs to be completely aware
of the ramifications of one's reactions
so the result isn't resented by the rest.

.

10. Special Cynic, (Clinic).

So you're the seventh son of a seventh son, born with a silver spoon. I'm the bastard son of a baron, boarding at Paddington pontoon. May we fight the foe, say "Here we go". When duty calls we'll dance at balls with Algernon the Unlikely, saying to Percy " Crikey, I've got the time to make her mine before we go to war".

The aristocracy and its whores always keeping scores, counting cash, getting pleasure from treasure. May you rule the waves and waive the rules when jewels are in jeopardy. So you're the divine daughter of a Dauphin, don't think it brings you kudos. I'm the kin of a king who conquered the continent, so may I say "Up yours". If I don't want to, I won't do the chores.
Also, if I may be so bold to have told the fold "give me the gold", then I have the courage to convey countesses in my carriage to Cannes.

We're all fake, like the phoney false films. The only one superior is the one who sits on his posterior, the canny Creator of the Cosmos. We are not God free.

.

11. A Piece on War and Peace

The contentious, contemptuous, conscientious objector was objected to by a corrupt, corpulent colonel for caring for carnivores and cannibals and everybody else, including the enemy, and for refusing to rent them asunder by bayonet or more esoteric methods of extinguishing their existence when war raged, or practising while peace prevailed.

The conchie, Victor, was a vegan, and voted variously for parties promoting an absence of hostilities in their manifestos. However, his chosen candidates and parties weren't always successful, and ones with warmongering ways sometimes won the elections, which was when the fat officer fired his salvo of slander against the violence-shy Victor, calling him a cowardly custard, too scared to scheme in fighting the foe, in a dream for saying no!

The legislature legislated law that allowed people of principle to be prosecuted and parcelled off to prison to cells with piss-pots and piss-poor conditions. But certain circumstances are only temporary, while evil episodes are judged and those involved punished eternally. So voices like Victor's will prevail, and Victor's will shall prevail despite gaol, hail, gale, wail this male and many more with his norms, values and mores shall assail the gates of Heaven and avail themselves of immortality, all things considered. It is necessary to add that protectors and defenders practising the minimum of violence are excused condemnation by the Lord and I, you'll be relieved to hear.

.

THE PREVIOUS ESSAYS OF A FORMER PARANOID SCHIZOPHRENIC

12. Thirty Years On

Miss April May June White-Brown-Green was second to take the minutes of the hours of daily meetings that went on weekly for months each year during the parliamentary sessions.

Ape, as she was affectionately known, was actually attracted to an actor appearing twice nightly at the Apollo Theatre.

They are about the same age, and Ape is about as attractive, for a woman, as Arthur the thespian is for a man, which helps. Both of them shared a similar upper-working class background spent in Essex, and their ambitions for the future are alike.

But there is a problem. The fact is that although Ape has attended the Apollo on numerous occasions to see Arthur in this latest production, usually after the adjournment of Parliamentary proceedings during the week, and he has witnessed her sitting near the front row of the theatre on these occasions, they have never been formally introduced, and have yet to meet.

They have just caught each other's eye. I know this because Ape mentioned to me one day that Arthur had either had something in his eye during the previous night's performance, or had winked at Ape, also knowing Ape and reading a bit about Arthur in the programme.

Being a cat-lover like both of them and also a hopeless romantic, not to say an interfering matchmaker, I decided I'd be the catalyst of their meeting, hopefully the start of a beautiful friendship, not to say love affair. I went with Miss W.B.G. to the Apollo during a recess of the House, and persuaded an albeit reluctant A.M.J. to visit Arthur's dressing-room subsequent to the performance which I enjoyed greatly; I know a wink when I see one, which we did.

Artie appeared overjoyed to meet April, in an understated way, and, after chit-chat about the show and his part in it, the course of true love flowed with the first of many an invitation from Arthur to Ape being made. She seemed shy, but assented on this first occasion, as she always did subsequently.

They now have three children and all five of them attended my funeral thirty years to the day after I'd introduced A. to A..

13. Not a Freud

My pet parrot ate a coffee-coloured carrot, consequently Ziegmund, for he was named thus, suffered stomach ache, at least that's what he seemed to say. This multi-coloured miracle of evolution looked off-colour so to speak, so off we trotted to the veterinary surgeon.

At the PDSA, for I get service there free, being on benefit, Chloe the vet examined Ziegmund and, using very advanced psychological techniques, diagnosed him as suffering from depression, with the belly-ache being just a symptom of this. The bird, normally an extrovert, had become inhibited, not having a Polly parrot to relate to, only my human household. Apparently he yearned for a parrot partner with whom to share everyday life, or at least that's what the educated Chloe suspected.

Having just received my Christmas bonus and financial assistance from my ex-partner, I withdrew what seemed an appropriate amount from my account, and took Ziegmund to the nearest pet shop, where we were introduced to two female parrots. He was initially interested in the prettier of the two, but soon realised that Genevieve, as she was called, thought a lot of herself, and obviously regarded Ziegmund as a loser, because of his depression.

The other bird looked beyond my parrot's present personal difficulties and saw that she, Xavier, could help Ziggy regain his normal outgoing personality and, in so doing, provide herself with a partner to be proud of.

Purchasing Xavier proved a problem, for the price was higher than I anticipated, but providence provided in the form of a postal order which had arrived in that morning's mail. I had it in my pocket, so, after leaving a deposit at the pet shop, I went to the post office and returned with the full amount, reuniting my parrot with his new love.

I was so relieved that I could supplement Xavier's purchase price with the proceeds of selling Ziegmund's previous, now deceased, mate for stuffing.

THE PREVIOUS ESSAYS OF A FORMER PARANOID SCHIZOPHRENIC

14. Lost

The portly prince in the principality palace conveyed a chalice, worth a pretty penny, to the chatty, chubby prelate in the chapel.

The ageing aristocrat arranged, as agreed, for the chap of the cloth to carry the chalice from the palace chapel to the Cathedral of St. Peter in Rome, for the Pope to perform communion on the feast day of the patron saint of astronauts and other assorted travellers, St Christopher, for whom he had affection due to the protection provided by the patient saint to the prince's pater and mater when they pursued panthers and other predatory creatures on the sunny Dark Continent early in the previous century.

The upper-class chip off the old king cared for those who dared despite being scared however they fared whenever they fought the foe without finding fault away they would go, and were handsomely rewarded by the Colonel-in-Chief, His Royal Highness, for their efforts.

The particular people earning enmity, the enemy, changed as the clocks chimed, causing confusion, but, having hate in their hearts and love only in their loins, it's no wonder that fighting starts after tossing coins .

Notable nobility nurtures peace, while people of poisoned personality persevere with warlike ways, wondering about winning while killing is losing.

15. The Item

Harriet Marriott made a request to borrow it now, as tomorrow it might be too late, but it was with sorrow it was deemed out of the question. Buddy Friend, Harriet's chum, will send a substitute for her consideration, should she convey concern sometime soon.

Miss Marriott's mate then provided a pair of winkle-pickers particularly suited for her purpose upon perceiving her need. But he still succeeded, and indeed did heed the greed, feed the seed and supply the mead to those who read and smoke the weed alas also.

Harriet wished to be dressed like the rest in her someday best when she becomes a guest at Buddy's behest at the Oktoberfest. Hence he woos with shoes and gets caressed when she was dressed the following evening.

With her long flowing fair hair and daringly plunging neckline seemingly without a care no-one glared, but they all stared as she fared finely, finally being paired with ruddy Buddy in big muddy boots, but he wasn't fuddy-duddy but fashionably polite, lifting her above puddles.

She gave a glance, he took the chance. So they did dance. They drank, into his arms she sank, all other men drew a blank. He won, he's her sun, she's his moon, he's her boon. They heard their tune, it will always mean this scene to them.

16. Not a Blot

U. Lott was a great chap, always thinking of others. If it was a question of putting himself out to do anyone a favour it was resolved in favour of that.

Unfortunately he took up with a woman, Y. Nott, who wasn't totally positive, just thinking of reasons she shouldn't do something, justifying inactivity.

It is with regret I report that the latter didn't extend to usually horizontal exertion, and a tot was born to Y. Nott and U. Lott after the usual preamble of courtship and intimacy had taken place.
This parental mismatch led to the baby, who incidentally was a boy with the biblical name of Lot, getting mixed messages about whether or not he should help others in need as he grew up. Luckily Lot had much mental ability and became prone to philosophising, weighing the pros and cons and ramifications of his putative actions prior to them.

Unlike his Dad, Lot would consider the cost and benefit to himself and the other party involved before agreeing to assist.

This prevented Lot being taken advantage of, as people thought twice before asking the calculating Lot to do anything for them. Whereas with U. Lott, his attitude was reciprocated with generosity and respect. Y. Nott just wasn't asked.

17. A Character of the Cosmos

Being concerned about consternation in our constellation I feel obliged to remind inhabitants that the goal is Heaven.

Bring about blessings for benediction, forget friction and fuss; surely one knows that being good now achieves our future target.

Forgiveness for transgressions is the correct form for and by ourselves and others; we can at least be this divine. Our duty is the dereliction of evil and the promotion of positive possibilities; every intention should be honourable.

Our thoughts, words, deeds and omissions are only initiated with our permission; we should be in control, and need to choose truth carefully.

Being unafraid of past, present and future reality leads to behaviour being correctly chosen. If one was in possession of complete knowledge of all, like God, one would be cool and calm.

This not yet being possible, faith of this should be engaged, then one will be assured of the wonder of our different worlds and eternity, together with future experience of them.

.

THE PREVIOUS ESSAYS OF A FORMER PARANOID SCHIZOPHRENIC

18. There Have Been

Pioneers prospecting, panning for precious gold
Blue-blooded bombardiers whose behaviour is bold
Ermine-skinned Eskimos whose actions are eccentric
Vicious geometrists whose circles are concentric
Genial jockeys jumping for joy
New mothers whose child is a boy

Discoverers discovering far distant lands
Musicians making melodies in fascinating bands
Housewives having hundreds of harrowing hours
Florists arranging their flowers in bowers
Workers reflexing on production lines
Schoolchildren studying cosines

Politicians posing and posturing in public
Publishers printing their lines in italic
Criminals considering their conspiracy
Pirates planning their piracy
Prelates praying for peace
Warriors wishing war would cease

Living a lifetime leave legacies that last
Invest in ideas whose influence is vast
Be as good and God-like as possible
Forget religion with miracles impossible
Seek salvation and save your soul
Head for Heaven, make that your goal.

19. The Exhibitors

The explorers expedited the exhibition of the expedition, which told tales of treks in torrid temperatures through terribly tough terrain. The display in detail of the destination, Djibouti, drove dozens to distraction, while others walked away wearily. Col. John Tennant-Pennant would tell attendees of the attention to all aspects of the intrinsic organisation of the entire affair, until even the most avid enthusiast suffered tiredness.

The Colonel and his constant companion Capt. Morgan, a rum fellow, always appeared refreshed, as if mounting this exhibition of exhibits of exhaustive research didn't exhaust but rather did invigorate them.

Corporal Punish meant well, but he hindered his comrades from the trip through his pugnacious proclivities. He had been trained to kill, and was spoiling for a fight with anyone he considered not quite appreciative enough of the show. Punish by name, punish by nature.

When Sid Crombie, a local skinhead, turned up sneering at the soldiers' achievements and leering at their partners, anything but puny Punish pushed Sid to one side and punched him on the other. Crombie reacted by head-butting the gallant Captain, who had stepped in to finish the fracas. Morgan fell in a heap at the Colonel's feet, while Punish was restrained by disciplined dogs of the

Salivation Army.   Soon he was led away and confined to barracks pending an investigation, while Sid continued to view examples of the Colonel's feats.

Unfortunately possible funders of further journeys found the unfavourable publicity connected with this unpleasant incident mitigated against the provision of further finance, thus punishing all for this demonstration of machismo by a man schooled in violence.

20. Mister M.

Mickey Mirth was a comical character, larger than life, all his life so far. He could be found buying a round in a bar or fooling around like a star, except when he was driving a car. In which case he stuck to tea totally enjoying sobriety, not that he had fear of a beer you understand, but he wouldn't have one in his hand even when listening to a band, when expecting to control a vehicle.

He wouldn't have one for a nickel or a penny, even with Jenny; in that case, he would think it base, and wouldn't be able to look a policeman in the face, not that there might be a chase, but he wouldn't act in haste.

He preferred to gain satisfaction through deferred gratification, containing his immediate desires to get the treasure of pleasure in future. Since his birth on Earth Mr. Mirth had made a stand, and planned to be as good as an angel, thinking of every angle he could before coming to a decision about what to achieve next.

He was seldom perplexed because he didn't leave anything to chance; his lot he enhanced continually, mentally and materially, not to mention in his relationships. He thought this only prudent, but it would be impudent to speculate that he was a control freak, for he was too meek, just seeking salvation through self-discipline.

THE PREVIOUS ESSAYS OF A FORMER PARANOID SCHIZOPHRENIC

His wealth was also in good humour; he could accept a tumour on a femur or an escaped puma or lemur with the same equanimity as someone treating him unequally, like a bully or a dim immature soul without an appropriate goal. And he liked fun and was funny, not that he got any money for it, but because it made everyone's day sunny when he told the one about the stoat on the boat and acted the goat.

There was no dearth of jokes and japes and worthy, wholesome merry-making, making it worth spending time with Mickey Mirth.

21. Hell and Heaven

The devil deliberately derelicts duty daily. Lucifer lacks enlightenment. Satan seeks and exploits weakness. St Nick gives in to feelings when true thoughts should be employed.
God gives guidance, the senses don't lie.

Knowledge derives from self-control; acknowledging facts leads to self-actualisation. Faith when in ignorance and patience in problem solving lead to stability, while determination combined with willpower and increasing strength contribute to solutions. Peace of mind, contentment and happiness are the result of thinking what you know and believe, enabling joy to be reaped. Nature is nurturing, and genuineness in human nature gives appreciation of the wonder and logic of all of the Lord's creation.

Truth is love and untruth is hate; people seek others with a similar perception of reality and dislike, and are threatened by, different views unknown to them personally. There is a unity in love between those who believe the truth of their experience, and suspicion and jealousy from liars whose unity is in hate and guilt and lessened by friction.

Be assured that Heaven awaits truth thinkers, while meanwhile life is pleasurable. For those not strong enough to think the truth and those weak enough to lie, their desires become undermined and perverted, rendering the results of their energy expenditure evil and their reward Hell.

22. Help

Jayne Elaine Payne met Lloyd-Floyd Freud-Boyde at the psychiatric outpatients' clinic on a sunny July Monday morning. Jayne, having problems, had sought assistance from her General Practitioner, Dr Proctor, who subsequently referred her here. Jayne, reliant on buses, had arrived early for her appointment and Lloyd-Floyd had found her by herself in an empty waiting room, where he began to talk to her about what had brought her here (not the buses but her specific problems).

Miss Payne initially found it difficult to relate her most intimate historical secrets to a complete stranger, but after overcoming her inhibitions went on at some length, which she found terrifically therapeutic. Unfortunately her reminiscences were interrupted when the psychiatrist, Dr Brain, called Mr Freud-Boyde into his 9.30am appointment.

Miss Payne had to wait another thirty minutes for her's.

23. Physical

Mary Milligan was a famous British porn star. She starred in films, magazines, books and revues in the 1970s when she was in her 20's. She performed all sorts of sexual activities, some of which must have upset her, explaining that everything is permissible, and equating this with freedom.

Unfortunately, she appears to have been labouring under a massive misapprehension about what she found acceptable and unacceptable, for she became more and more desperately unhappy, and eventually killed herself by taking an overdose of drugs. There are right things to do with one's body, and then again wrong things. Right things equate with love and goodness, and wrong things obviously with hate and badness.

Each of us knows instinctively the difference, and, if one is wisely trying to achieve what we all truly want, one uses one's body for right, love and goodness in a similar way to one's mind. Thus this is the freedom we have, to self-actualise (fulfil one's innate aims and satiate one's desires) or be destructive, not fulfilling one's positive potential, which, you will agree, is a waste.

24. The Cost

Grant Forsyth-Smythe met Hugh Pugh outside Titton Conservative Club; they were both on the membership committee, with a view to having a brain-storming session on the different ways that new members could be attracted to their club. With the party nationally floundering after the Chancellor's budget, this was proving a difficult task.

Grant and Hugh decided to concentrate on the social aspects of the club, which are considerable, and to pay less attention to the politics and policies they stand for. Going into the club that morning they were shocked to see Bill Hill, a former leading light of the club, who had recently been found guilty of embezzlement, chatting up Flossy the cleaner. They slyly avoided Bill on their way to the committee room, where they met Harry Barry and Lex Bex.

The latter two both agreed with the strategy Grant and Hugh had adopted to emphasize the social aspects of the club rather than any beliefs, values or aims involved. They all agreed to invite Ashley Bashley and Horace and Doris Morris of the social activity committee along to the next meeting.

Meanwhile bossy Flossy, the cleaner, came to the door, emphasising that the room needed cleaning and it needed cleaning now. So they adjourned. The thing about achievement is that it takes many, many co-ordinated steps over a sustained period of time to come about. What Grant, Hugh, Harry and Lex realised is that what seems a side-effect of the Conservative Clubs, namely the election of that party, is really the prime purpose and all the most successful socialising in the world cannot justify such an outcome.

.

25. Fame

We have all heard about the lady that sticks out from the herd. I speak of Lady O'Grady, the cattle baron O'Grady's spouse. Lady O'Grady, or to use her professional name, Carly Varley, was either a tiger or a pussy on the catwalk, according to whatever was required in her role as a top international supermodel. She also graced the pages of glossy magazines everywhere on Earth.

Since the birth of her son Harley, Carly has worked less and taken motherhood as seriously as a thriving social life dictates. Flitting from one home near Fray Bentos, Argentina, to a Mediterranean hideaway, on to London and then North America, is not unusual during her busy monthly schedule. Our heroine is to be admired for her battle against the use of drugs in the fashion industry, lending her name as patron or matron to several society charities established for this purpose in England and abroad. She is also known as a prominent vegetarian, protesting that "Meat is Murder", despite her husband's involvement in that industry. Indeed, she boasts that every unit of currency she spends is blood-free, coming from her own earnings rather than Lord O'Grady's gravy, much to the chagrin of the Dowager Lady O'Grady, who enjoys Jamaican bacon and pork chops as well as karate.

Carly insists that her husband is the only man she has ever loved, the father of Harley, and defends his right to choose, just as long as he does not expect her to cook parts of animals' bodies or eat them herself, while Harley eats a little paltry poultry, perhaps twice a week. The rumours of a romance between our main subject and Zero Sun, the failed Japanese Kamikaze pilot turned chopstick tycoon, are much exaggerated, and only those of poisoned mind could doubt the affirmation of the voice of sincere integrity, that of the Honourable Harley Varley's mother.

I believe that the reporter C. Lyon is lying all down the line and maybe getting himself in deep water, by communicating differently.

26. Regrets and Repentance

Captain William Kidd (1645-1701) and the Buccaneers played for the English off the North American coast. As a reward for his sterling service Bill was granted a Royal Commission to suppress outlaws at sea in the Indian Ocean in 1695. However, Pirate Records centred in Madagascar seemed to offer him a better deal, and he joined them, raising the Jolly Roger and downing galleons of beer.

Going back to Boston was a big mistake, as he was promptly arrested and returned to England, where the fact he had represented that country against the French was forgotten, and the only stage he saw was a gallows where he was executed in 1701. It is a matter of conjecture as to how justified it was to kill him on that stage at that stage. There is still doubt about the justice of his conviction, but it is my conviction and that of many of sound mind that capital punishment, in the capital or elsewhere, is counter-productive and leads to dead villains being worshipped as heroes subsequent to their demise. Also, they are denied the opportunity to regret what they have sung and repent. What became of his band, the Buccaneers, is not recorded, and there is nothing on DVD either.

27. Sickness, Recreation and Desperation

Shirley Hurley-Burley was involved in a confused, crowded confrontation in a town precinct shop with Derek Eric Cedric Frederick, an impatient, irritable and unpleasant senior citizen, when it was unclear whose turn it was to be served next in the bookies.

Shirley is a middle-aged woman in the kind of ill-health that prevents her working. Her main hobby is watching the sport of kings on her television, often having a small flutter to increase her interest and level of excitement and involvement in the activity. On this particular Wednesday she spotted Derek, a visitor to the area, and recognised him as a stranger and was a bit nervous of him because of his dishevelled, unkempt appearance, which was the result of years of dependence on the demon drink and little input of love and care from himself towards himself or anyone else, or anybody else towards him.

Consequently short of cash, Mr Frederick was desperate for a win on the gee-gees with a view to financing a desperate craving for alcohol. Convinced he had chosen a long-odds winner for the next race, he rushed to place the bet with the bookmaker's cashier and collided with the patiently waiting Shirley, who was unusually betting on a subject other than horse racing, though with her usual low stake money.

Derek, convinced Shirley had pushed in, fussed and fumed, muttering under his breath, furious that he might not have time to place his bet while this woman wasted her time betting the second baby would be called " Casanova" Beckham.

This upset Shirley, who subsequently was not cheered up, even when the horse Derek had just managed to get a bet on came last in the field. But Shirley was resilient and surely recovered soon, having the strength that comes from responding appropriately to suffering.

Derek stayed in a foul mood until he collected his pension and bought drink.

28. Regrets

Killer-Man Jarro is the tallest boxer on the continent of Africa. He has defeated lots of the world's most celebrated social climbers. That is, boxers who have advanced from poverty to an acceptably elaborate standard of living, moving mountains to obtain the dizzy heights of a penthouse in Paris complete with penthouse pets, or a villa near Venice and all stops in between.

Killer-Man was obviously commensurately rewarded for his feats with his fists, making his defeated opponents' financial achievements look like chickenfeed or penthouse pet food. Financially astute until one unfortunate blow to the head, the fortune of Jarro marches on, now in the hands of well paid advisers who risk only their reputation for integrity, not damage to their brains.

No longer able to box cleverly, K-M is surrounded by hangers-on in the form of an extensive entourage, and has obligations to ex-wives and his several children. But his fortune isn't increasing, even by the current rate of inflation, once his expenses and their extravagance has been taken care of. Nevertheless, he insists in his lucid moments that he wouldn't do or have done anything differently if he had his time again, except for blocking the blow that bludgeoned his brain.

29. Rock Around the Clock

There were two female friends named Kay Bright-Day and Gaye Darke-Knight who never ceased weekly clubbing. On one particular occasion they met two brothers, Ray and Wayne Light.

It was an enlightening experience for all of them when Ray and Wayne spoke to Kay and Gaye under the spotlights of the club 'Diva'. Soon they retired to a quieter area away from the dance floor, by a table near the upstairs bar, where they became engrossed in each other's company, Kay and Ray, then Gaye and Wayne, to the exclusion of many others still on the pull. For these four had met their sole soul-mates with whom they would achieve their many goals and share their fates during their lives' future dates, finally passing Heaven's Gates. But I am being premature.

Existence on this planet brings its duties and responsibilities to oneself, one's family, one's friends, one's society, and last and certainly not least the Lord. Being tentatively spiritual people, all four of the aforementioned decided on marriage with a carriage taking them on a, in Kay and Ray's situation, pilgrimage to Lourdes, with a view to restoring Kay's lung function as she suffered with asthma, and, in Gaye and Wayne's case, a tour of the violent holy land where they both prayed for the restoration of Kay's health, their carriage being an air carriage.

THE PREVIOUS ESSAYS OF A FORMER PARANOID SCHIZOPHRENIC

These two separate honeymoons began after a double-wedding in the summer, eighteen months after they had met each other's future life-long lovers for the first time. Both holidays went well and boded superbly for the future, as these were true loves.

Kay Bright-Day-Light found enough strength after many years of struggle to give up the weed, and immediately her asthma diminished. Thenceforth all four enjoyed good health, and used the security and certainty this brings to start families, but only after they had gained a measure of career success that they subsequently continued after the babies came along until the different days on which they retired.

The Bright-Day-Lights and the Darke-Knight-Lights led contented lives with the peace of mind that good moral standards allow.

30. Heroes

'Royal' Tex 'The King' Rex had been associated with Rebecca 'Becs' Rex for four years longer than they had been married. In addition to the attraction that these red-blooded heterosexuals share for each other, and the specific activity during which it manifests itself, i.e. Tex and Becs' enjoy sex, they also share passions for Elvis Aaron Presley and the British blue-blooded Royal Family.

It isn't that they admire the Windsors' singing and Elvis' moral leadership, but rather vice-versa. Not that there is anything wrong with the way the Windsors carry a tune, but their broadcasts usually stick to speech, whilst Mr Presley concentrated in particular on performing songs until his untimely death at a reasonably young age in 1977.

Despite their rather primitive choices of role-models, Tex and Becs have the kind of non-judgemental attitude that allows them to put E.A.P. on a pedestal in spite of his moral shortcomings which were much publicised at the time of his death; you may remember gluttony, drug-taking, alcohol abuse and sexual deviations being mentioned.

Some people consider that talent makes a person special, in spite of obvious deficiencies in maturity, holiness, innocence or goodness. Well I for one would rather spend time with someone who has made the right intellectual choices in terms of good and bad, than someone who has demonstrated weakness in decision making, choosing wrong, no matter how talented that individual may be in some direction.

Do we mistake being good at something in particular with being good through and through? I consider that each person must be judged for their complete being.

31. The Why

Felix Stowe was in his gap year after a public school career at Stowe. He worked with Stevie Door at the docks in Felixstowe prior to attending the local university, where he plans to study all aspects of popular music culture since its inception in the early 1950s.

His interest in this particular subject had been stimulated many years previously by his music-mad mater and pop-fan pater, and encouraged by them ever since. But it's not only the culture that turns young Felix on; in the creation and the performance of the music itself the 18 year old has been gifted with talent, and will spend about half of his time continuing to learn how to sing, play the bass guitar and write melodies and lyrics.

A busy time ahead for the lad, but meanwhile he is learning about the real world while saving with his temporary employment at the docks. His father wants him to be grounded with an insight and appreciation into the world of the working classes who, after all, will be purchasing his products for many years to come, guaranteeing him a prosperous livelihood if they find them pleasing.

So far, as young Felix reported to his parents, he has found his work-mates' main preoccupation to be the fortunes of their particular choice of football team. A secondary interest is pop music, with females coming a close third. Conversation about mobile phones is also common.

His middle class background gave him certain assumptions which he is revising, about what is worthwhile spending time on, while his work colleagues have different assumptions, pickled by the alcohol they are always imbibing.

Felix's ideals are controlling his behaviour, and include a belief in truth, right, strength, goodness, love and beauty being the basis of a good life. He is coming across conduct derived from untruth, wrong, weakness, badness, hate and ugliness, and learning that some people have entirely the wrong idea about life and God. In the revision of his assumptions it's implicit that some have made many mistakes and need forgiveness, which is divine. What happened to Felix I don't know.

32. H.T.P.D.

Heaven's Thought Police Department, England Country Division.

As you know, we were established by God to monitor the behaviour of Earthlings, which is directed by their thought reaction to their previous experience. We were given the power, which we use constantly, to affect the emotions and feelings of the individual in relation to their thoughts.

Thus if people think/decide to be good we will make them feel good, and likewise if they think/decide to be bad we will make them feel bad. So their entire range of response is complete; they shall be good or they shall be bad. People who sit on the fence will suffer until they decide on one path or the other.

People's behaviour will be derived from these decisions, and the results of their time on Earth will be according to this behaviour. It may be said that we are encouraging badness by making some individuals feel bad, but it is immutable in humans that they like feeling/being good and hate feeling/being bad, so by making them feel bad we are making an effort to motivate them to improve and decide to become good.

In order to effect such change in these people a fair amount of time on Earth shall have been allotted to them, as it shall be for those who've decided to be good early on to achieve appropriate results.

THE PREVIOUS ESSAYS OF A FORMER PARANOID SCHIZOPHRENIC

"What of those who don't get much time on Earth?" I hear you say. That is the subject for another essay yet to come. Meanwhile, have faith.

33. Cruising

Most people know that British shipping lines are taking on foreign nationals as crew to reduce costs, as they are paid less than their British counterparts. What is little known is that Sammy Singh-Song, a half-Bangladeshi half-Chinese crooner, has such a great talent that he is rewarded commensurately to such an extent that Honor and Conor O'Connor, sister and brother of that all-round entertainer Les O'Connor, complain to anyone who will listen that their sibling is comparatively underpaid when both are employed on cruise ships in the Caribbean.

To be fair, it should be pointed out that Les jokes about this situation and freely admits that Sammy sings superbly with a vocal range from that of Tiny Tim (remember 'Tiptoe through the Tulips') to the remarkable Louis Armstrong, Satchmo, 'Wonderful World' himself. Les asserts that while Samuel is tremendously gifted in this department he, himself, has talents in different directions as well, such as interviewing, presenting, and comedy. These varied skills guarantee that Les shall never be idle, while Sammy's only speciality of performing songs could saturate the market, possibly having a soporific effect on the audience, perhaps leading him to enforced spells of unemployment.

Les explains this regularly to Honor and Conor, who choose not to listen.

34. The Scarlet Jacket

Bruce Brewster kept a ruddy rooster on his farm in Devizes near the Assizes. On an occasion well-remembered, a hungry felon who had escaped from custody and who was well practised in butchery (and having no custard) had taken Rudolph the ruddy rooster prisoner, with a view to plucking and preparing him for consumption at the rear of the farm outbuildings out of sight of the honest farm labouring types and Bruce himself.

The gallant rooster was having none of this unconvicted criminal's intent, and making as much noise as he could, he alerted Bruce's son, Dexter Brewster, to his present predicament and the possible particular fate that might befall him, in this way. Dex, realising something was really wrong with Rudolf, grabbed his shotgun from it's locked metal cabinet and, enlisting aid from his father's employees, shot off in the direction of the squawks and high-pitched shrieks.

They soon found Casper Jasper Barrington, a local businessman who had been recently charged with fraud, desperately trying to silence Rudolf, alas too late to save himself. Dexter and his father's men carried out a citizen's arrest of this former master of the hunt, who, without his dogs, found a chicken too brave an adversary.

35. At The Red Lion, (Karaoke Fact).

The King and Queen of Karaoke in their particular suburb at this time summoned all those loyal to them and performed their party pieces promptly from early evening until closing time.

There was Queen Kirstie cavorting, bumping and grinding and strutting her stuff whilst singing her songs. Her female followers, the friends, cheered and shouted encouragement as she did her routine, which was anything but routine, and involved using part of the pub furnishings, fixtures and fittings in a way that the men found fascinating and stimulating.

Her King this night had a Louis Armstrong feel from the tunes he sang to the way he sang, but the way he put his songs over with body language was eclipsed by the royal drinker of vodka and orange, Kirstie.

The crowd was extensive on this Saturday evening, 8th September 2008, with two ladies' birthdays being celebrated, one of them the Queen's friend, Pat, the other held in a small, much quieter group. There were the regular drinkers and karaoke fans, and lots of not very strange strangers' faces apparent.

It has been suggested in recent times that this Saturday night had a certain joie de vivre, a je ne sais quoi that left the following few weeks feeling empty and unexciting by comparison.

THE PREVIOUS ESSAYS OF A FORMER PARANOID SCHIZOPHRENIC

Certainly the absence of the louder birthday group, comprising as it does of attractive ladies, I name Claire as an example, who know how to uninhibitedly have a good time within the bounds of decency, led to at least one man looking forward to seeing them again. I should know, for he is the author of this piece.

36. Her Choice, (Karaoke Fiction).

Anything but silly Billy and Lily Dilley dallied, drinking Drambuie delicately during the dancing, while Andy and Sandy Ghandi, the King and Queen of Karaoke Kapers, and their princesses Candy and Mandy Ghandi, ran the show superbly.

Then soon, with her inhibitions loosened by the liqueur, Lily began cavorting, bumping and grinding while strutting her stuff, singing her songs including 'Cold Turkey', encouraged by fellow revellers at this Boxing Day function. Her friends and female fans and followers in this suburb at the time cheered and shouted encouragement as she did her routine, which was anything but routine and involved using parts of the pub furnishings, fixtures and fittings in a way the men found both fascinating and stimulating. Lily is one foxy filly.

Billy was super at singing Sinatra songs in a similar manner to the master himself, but the way he put his lyrics over with body language was eclipsed by his partner in Drambuie drinking, Lily. The Dilleys and the senior Ghandis went back a long way to the rear of the Royal Red Cross Keys garden at about 10pm, while Candy and Mandy maintained momentum with the marvellous music, making minutes speed like seconds.

William and Lily, Andrew and Sandra briefly braved the winter cold in a bid to bring privacy to these particular proceedings, which involved congratulations to all four for the upcoming announcement of the forthcoming engagement of Billy and Lily's son, Willy, to Andy and Sandy's daughter, Candy. The toast was in champagne, as the parents planned who was to say what to the crowd, which consisted of the regular drinkers and karaoke fans, and lots of strange and not very strange faces apparent in the pub on this festive occasion.

It was soon decided that Mandy might be most appropriate to tell the patrons the families' news, as she and her sister are so close. Mandy concurred, and within moments did the deed.
The short speech produced cheers and a certain joie de vivre was engendered, a celebratory je ne sais quoi that I cannot quite put my finger on.

However, suffice it to say that Mandy is still single, and more than one man of good taste intends to change this situation if and when the opportunity arises.

37. Fervour Fever

Sapphire Ruby Diamond, whose given name was Joan Precious Stone, is the lead singer and drummer in the band, "The Four Degrees". Blue Gene Buttons plays the organ, while Darren Barron is on bass guitar and Anton Danton concentrates on lead guitar, with occasional vocal forays.

Most of the audiences at their recent gigs would agree, who wouldn't, that any band with, coincidentally, a similar name is one degree under by comparison, when it comes to singing songs simulating stimulation. Indeed the 'Fantastic Four', as their fans refer to them, seem so supersonically satisfied that psychiatrists seeing their stagecraft have suggested that they are somewhat high.

Beryl Cheryl Terrill, the band's manager and self-publicist, denies that they drink alcohol to excess, drop drugs or smoke dope, insisting instead that adrenalin only assists their hippy happy-go-lucky hours of hip-hopping, harnessing harmonious vibes culled from the ramblings of their guru, Maharishi Mahesh Yogi Bear of Delhistone Park.

It is well known that the Maharishi's cult regards the Red Bull as sacred. Could this be the explanation for the immense energy input and expenditure evident in these entertainers' evening exertions and post-performance parties?

We perhaps have a possible right to know.

38. Freedom and Captivity

I would suggest that there is a correlation between truth; right; strength; goodness; love; beauty; happiness; and Heaven. Furthermore, that there is a correlation between untruth; wrong; weakness; badness; hate; ugliness; misery; and Hell.

Those who are afraid that knowing, thinking and believing any particular truth, in case it has a detrimental effect on them i.e. kills them, makes them homosexual or lesbian or perverted, mad, unhappy, makes them lose a sense or senses, unable to read, write, remember, talk, move, mentally damaged or change their desire to be good, or makes them effect these things on other people, will be driven to a life embracing deeds, thoughts and words of the second of my correlations.

Whereas, if they are confident of accepting the truth totally, the more the better, then they shall be fulfilled in life and death, as described in my first correlation.

39. Taken for Granted

Douglas I O' Man, Beverley Hills and Winifred 'Win' Chester are partners in the firm of international estate agents 'Anytime, Anyplace Ltd'. They are able to enable anyone with the necessary wherewithal to rent or buy any size estate anywhere in the world.

From coastal resorts on the Mojave Sea or Birmingham Islands to inland locations, such as Canary City or Greenwich Village, properties are made available. Operating from plush offices in New Chicago, St Peterscow, Shangjing and Clovelly amongst other big cities, Dougie, Bev and Win employ the cream of professionals in that industry worldwide, planning to expand in the near future.

Their offices are amongst the most luxuriously appointed, and the Rolling Stones' 'Abbey Road' and 'Please, Please Me' albums are only a couple of examples of Mozart's work, piped along with the discreet air-conditioning on a seven days a week opening schedule.

Willy B Willoughby is only one of hundreds of satisfied customers, having purchased a penthouse cellar from 'Anytime, Anyplace Ltd' only two weeks ago.

He says "I was at a loss to know where to locate my home, as property is dearer in the south;

THE PREVIOUS ESSAYS OF A FORMER PARANOID SCHIZOPHRENIC

Reykjavik, Niceland seemed ideal, as it is situated midway between North America and Europe, and fish is so cheap there. Also, I now have an outhouse where I can house visiting friends and relatives away from the frightening November 5th Gunpowder Plot celebrations, which incidentally distress my pet cat, Rover".

Now you may find the above nonsensical, but it does illustrate to one how much a new arrival on the planet Earth has to learn in terms of names of things, including geography and popular culture.

Lest we forget, we start with knowledge of nothing but our desires, and even these may be misinterpreted by ourselves and others.

Do appreciate your capacity for learning and personal growth.

40. A Contribution

Detective Inspector Vincent Ince knew the Rev Christian Church and Canon Ball from the shooting club they all attended, but was still surprised to see them at the bar mitzvah of Bernie, the son of the president of the club, Joshua Gatling-Remington-Colt, whose father incidentally won the George Cross in Korea. Some said he only acted bravely to get the pension associated with that gallantry award, but I believe his action was instinctive, stemming from a courageous character.

At this celebration of Bernie's coming of age were guests, obviously including relatives, from all strata of local society, but they had one thing in common; they all wanted to see Bernie grow into an upright, God-fearing citizen with a social conscience, but this seemed to be a forlorn hope as V. Ince, or, to be more informal, Vince knew.

For Bernie had an addictive personality; habits of his included glue-sniffing (although some say there are worse things you can sniff), playing gaming machines, albeit illegally, anti-social behaviour while under the influence of glue, and thieving to finance his gambling.

But, as Chris Church and his friend in faith 'Billy' Ball knew from their work with the victim support scheme, Bernie, when confronted with the consequences of his crime, really regretted his wrong-doing and was very remorseful, which accounted for the leniency he was shown by the authorities including D.I. V.I. after he was caught.

The social inquiry reports following remarked upon the trauma suffered by Bernie when his mother was killed in a car accident. It was particularly terrible as he had been at a tender age, ten years old, when this had happened, and Bernie had been considerably closer to his mother than he was to any other mortal being.

So compassion and understanding were extended to the culprit, and psychological interventions, including bereavement counselling, were to be the order of the day. Bernie acknowledged his need for these and, years later, after regaining a healthy psyche and studying social sciences, made a significant contribution to his community in his career role as a psychiatric social worker.

Sometimes adversity, although damaging in the short-term, when fought and overcome, especially with others' assistance, can lead to considerable personal insights and development, engendering a helpful disposition and informed integrity, enabling its commission.

41. Ambition

The character Joseph Veal, when himself, Joe Veal, was usually jovial. However, since changing his name when he became an actor he seems to have lost his panache. His raison d'etre now is to make his assumed identify, Saul Ball-Hall-Paul, a star, and it seems he will go to any lengths to do this, but will it bring the rewards he is expecting?

Fame, fortune and influence, since being attained, have caused him nothing but grief. From being constantly harassed by the paparazzi and the public, to being ripped off by his banker and getting involved with partisan politicians who used him for their own ends, he feels nobody wants him for himself.

But, being a saleable commodity just didn't sit right with the historically jovial Saul B-H-P, and he began to aim for a life away from the spotlight. So, consolidating his remaining wealth, he returned from his Hollywood haunts and auditioned, just like anyone else, for the Royal Shakespeare Company. Being competent at his craft brought him considerable kudos. After being accepted by this company and carrying off different roles of many multifaceted personalities he earned the respect of his peers, not to say a living wage.

His standard of living decreased, but this was far outweighed by the increase in his quality of life. He found that when not working he had the opportunity to think and reflect upon figures he had met, as well as fictitious creations, and this engendered wisdom which he endeavoured to pass on while lecturing to drama students and others interested.

Since coming from California this chap had resumed calling himself his given name, Joe Veal, and pursued and maintained peace of mind.

42. Opinion

The Rev. Bulpitt was in the pulpit spouting bullshit. Why does the church, with its emphasis on truth, continue to insist that fantasy magic miracles were materialised by a mere mortal man, when everybody knows that miracles are impossible?

God created all, then left us to our own devices to be judged on our decisions and choices.
As if life isn't hard enough, they try to persuade those needing guidance that acts that couldn't possibly have happened as described are the literal truth. It's like, to get the church's approval we need to believe untruth.

We must choose the right decision based upon goodness, not necessarily expedience. In order to make an informed decision we need to have the complete facts and not be deluded by any fictions.

No human being has been or is a deity, and no deity has existed on Earth. Deities inhabit Heaven. I am willing to bet my eternal life on the above.

43. Animals

Sir Wayne Duane Swain's fortunes were on the wane. His ancestors had made a packet from swine who looked after and slaughtered pigs. This was in England, obviously, not Israel.

For these employees, (the swine), wanted little but food, wine and different alcohol, as they lived, for the most part, in tied cottages. While some socialised in cottages, most used the local pub, which, in addition to the pig farms, were owned by the Swain family.

So the Swains profited from low wages, high-priced pork, and alcoholism. Some say they exploited people, pigs and pubs. But, to look at this situation from their point of view, they provided employment, sustenance and social venues in deprived rural areas.

Incidentally, if you are a connoisseur of pork scratchings, you should look out for 'Swain's Rind' as it has a blinding taste and texture.

Wayne Swain, born in affluent circumstances, was knighted for services to polo, which costs a mint at the best of times. Sir Wayne had more losing streaks since winning the All England Polo Challenge Cup than his finest quality back-rashers had streaks, but this didn't diminish his enthusiasm for the sport, which he promoted personally publicly provincially and through printed publicity throughout the kingdom, including the principality of Wales.

You may wonder why I call pig farmers 'swine'. Perhaps I am over-reacting, as pigs are so intelligent, but think of care-home staff slaughtering their residents for consumption at the dinner table. In other words, mustn't the care given to pigs be totally insincere, as it is purely provided with a view to financial gain when the fattened pigs' lives are prematurely ended? How can the swine look pigs in the eye?

44. Kudos for Caring

Lola Zola was married to Jomo Como by Father Ramon Roman after a terrifically torrid time of romance led to love, leading to this lifelong commitment. At the reception the teetotal Lola drank cola, while Jomo asked his major-domo for a polar-cold glass of champagne prior to cooling off in the indoor solar-heated swimming pool, the jewel in the crown of his town residence, which is fit for a president's presence and was a wedding present from his parents, who are rather particular.

There was nothing peculiar about the latter pair, which prompted J.C. to act appropriately affectionately, according to mores and morals manifesting munificence towards the lovely, loving Lola on the occasion of their honeymoon, as well as prior to this and after it, until their ultimate day together many years later.

During their marriage they shared many interests, for instance, a love of nature, people, art, literature and music, and passed these enthusiasms and a zest and appetite for living as well as a sense of humour onto their offspring.

Indeed, the whole family was so well-balanced they could all have been tightrope walkers, and indeed the circus and other public spectacles were frequented and sometimes organised by them. Certainly, one year, Jomo's regatta was attended by Jomo Kenyatta, a gentleman and politician, and another event, Lola's skating championship, was attended by an ex-Bay City Roller. They got involved in these activities altruistically, attempting to raise filthy lucre for pure purposes such as protecting porpoises and persuading police to prosecute people who promoted pretences and who purported policies that could actually cut investors' income were praiseworthy. So it is evident that all sorts of services were supplied to society in a series seldom seen before or since by these spiritually beautiful beings.

They would simply say that it is love's legacy that is laudable in life, and give credit to the Creator. As this is correct I compliment them for coming to that conclusion.

45. A Fling or …

Saul-Paul Saulet-Paulet knew Paris Harris from the sixth-form at King Edward VI School. They had a ball as a rule in the university holidays, when they became reunited working at the Croft Tavern. They were good friends and sexually uninvolved with each other, although they were both vigorously attracted to different members of the opposite sex who, unfortunately, were already spoken for.

So they commiserated with each other over their thwarted desires and ambitions, and this drew them closer together when they went to 'New York, New York', a night club in Southampton, with a crowd after a busy Friday evening shift at the pub.

Being young and only fairly recently introduced to the dangerous delights of alcohol, they overdid their imbibing to such an extent that satiating their sexual needs seemed an excellent idea when the opportunity arose while both were staying the night at the home of a friend of Saul-Paul's, near the city centre, as the friend's parents were away and unable to 'interfere'.

Indeed the parents, Jean and Sean Frean, did unwittingly help in the commission of the acts of intercourse, as it was their condoms that were used by the couple. Mr and Mrs Frean would have been only too happy to oblige in the provision of the said condoms if they had knowledge of the circumstances, realising the risks that were being run.

Paris was enlightened, and expected little change in her relationship with S-P. However, Saul-Paul felt that things had developed and that he now had a 'claim' on Paris. This upset the girl, whose luck changed when the teenager she originally fancied madly split up with his girlfriend and chatted Paris up in the bar when she was working. She responded according to her feelings and arranged to meet him later.

Saul-Paul, aware of this, handled the situation extremely badly by leaving his bar job at the Croft and sending Paris unwise texts on his mobile phone. Their friendship had finished. It was over forever.

46. Hero-Worship

June E Clooney-Mooney-Rooney soon swooned upon hearing a tune played by Jake Cake-Lake-Wake, who would take any listener and make that person feel he was performing for their sake only, and that his lyrics about love were intended for them alone. But, unlike June, most did not go out of their way to discover the reality behind Jake's image.

June herself went to every gig of his within a hundred miles of her home town, wrote to this, her hero, regularly, spent her holidays commuting between outside his Weybridge residence and his London agent's office to meet him as he came and went, and, after many brief encounters and short conversations, liked to think she had a relationship with him, that he was a sincere, genuinely nice guy who replied to her letters personally in a way specifically special to her and nobody else.

In other words, she discovered that Jake's ability in music to reach out to the individual was just an extension of his true personality and character, as his off-stage behaviour demonstrated.

It wasn't until she became much older that she realised that Jake regarded women besides herself as unique too, and related to them in a similar way as he did to her. She could see that she had been a little naïve to think that his responses towards her were prompted by anything more than the flattery of her hero-worship and his pleasure in this.

Possibly this may be rather shallow.

47. Two True

Gerry and Kerry Berry-Ferry-Perry knew Callum Cullen-Mullen-Pullen from their local pub 'The Londonderry Arms'. Their son, Terry, regularly got merry there with Callum, both of them being in their early twenties, prior to going clubbing at the seafront. It was an unusual occasion when they failed to pull, and Terry and Callum became very sullen in their cups or, should I say, pint glasses, when the passes they made at lasses met with unresponsiveness.

However, this didn't deter the lads who were veterans in this, their chosen leisure pastime and pursuit, and the following weekend they were at it again. They knew pleasure speaking with two young ladies, Mary Carey and Sally O'Malley, who had recently started sharing the flat near 'The Londonderry Arms' where all four returned after the club they'd met in closed at two o'clock.

The girls were old-fashioned and endearingly respectable, and after coffees expected Terry and Callum to leave. The chaps became bemused by this peculiar development, and endeavoured to retain their self-esteem by arranging to 'phone Mary and Sally the next day in a bid to establish a rapport with repartee and charm.

The 'phone calls produced a plan to meet at the aforementioned pub that evening. Terry and Mary clicked, while Call and Sall eventually found each other boring, and only practised mutual toleration out of consideration for their friends. However, as the pub shut at 10.30pm on this Sunday, C and S didn't have to put up with each other for a very extended period, and politely wished each other "Goodnight" with relief.

Terry and Mary, on the other hand, quickly became smitten, and Terry couldn't wait to introduce Mary to Gerry and Kerry, his dad and mum, who entered the pub in time for 'Last Orders'. Mary made such a marvellous impression that the parents invited her to dinner the following day. Mary liked Mr and Mrs Berry-Ferry-Perry from the outset, and agreed to attend their three-bedroom terraced house in time for tucker, 7 o'clock, on the Monday. The three B-F-P's became fast friends with Mary, and it seemed to Terry that Mary was the girl made for him, and that if he missed this opportunity all his hopes of happiness in the future might disappear.

Within a week Terry proposed matrimony to Mary, who promised an answer within a month. Three weeks later, given a positive reply, Terry was momentarily euphoric and temporarily terrifically thrilled. Although able to act independently and always self-sufficient, Terry wanted to share his life and love with Mary whom he found beautiful, the acme of attractiveness for him; talented, intelligent, caring, sincere, genuine and truthful. While Mary felt likewise about Terry.

THE PREVIOUS ESSAYS OF A FORMER PARANOID SCHIZOPHRENIC

Although Terry had been a 'man about town' and 'played the field' like 'men of the world' do, he knew real love when it transpired, and wasn't so foolish as to let it pass him by.

48. Of Good Family

Clarence and Clarice Carruthers quickly created a couple of characters who they came to consider quite charming, called Claribel and Clarissa, obviously initially babies growing into gorgeous girls, well-groomed with golden hair and gentle temperaments.

Claribel was the tallest of these three Carruthers females when she was twenty-two years of age, whilst Clarissa was the most buxom, yet their mother possessed a certain wisdom that they wouldn't have for a couple of decades to come, which made the girls and their father admire her immensely.

Clarence possessed pride in his family, though no conceit, and was anxious that ambition to achieve be instilled into these individuals, so as to promote significant contributions to society from them.

The four Carruthers were always motivated morally to make maximum use of their abilities to do their best in every area, and this was demonstrated in their educational attainments and subsequent careers and success in their hobbies and interests.

This striving to be as good as possible gave them the strength when they faced adversity, difficulty and problems, to overcome the strife and resolve the issues satisfactorily. Their mutual support was of inestimable value to each of them, and continued until they all gained the places with God in Heaven that they came to deserve.

49. Maybe the M.-C.

Able Seaman Sidney Surrey's superiors sustained sight of seven seas being sailed splendidly by some seventy schooners. Certainly one Sunday soon S. Surrey saw something strange, as several civilians' statements seem to substantiate. As in the circumstances boasting beyond belief didn't become sensible Sid, a quest to establish with certainty what Sid had seen was commenced.

Civil Cecil and sad Cecilia Smith contended they had confronted the captain of Sid's ship, the "S.S. Finger", evidently with evidence which evoked empathy amongst almost the entirety of the courtroom auditorium's audience. To wit, these passengers reported perceiving Surrey strolling the deck of the vessel in question and apparently suffering shock, perhaps seeing nobody at all on board besides himself, as Sid had said.

Freddie Fish, captain of the Finger, confirmed the Smiths' evidence and argued that the salvage was legal and Sid Surrey sane and law-abiding. He further argued that six sailors who brought the salvaged vessel to port had, like Surrey before them, found no one on board, dead or alive, and no proof of any wrongdoing, as they would confirm themselves in due course.

To cut a long story short, the owners of the Finger were awarded salvage money for the vessel recovered by their ship, and prize-money was distributed by them to their crew and Sidney Surrey's widow. Any talk of a curse is idle speculation.

50. Chatting

Judy Moody was the speech therapist enlisted to assist Rebecca Pilkington-Pinkerton-Wilkinson overcome her vocal impediment.

Judy knew from her own personal experience that speech defects could have a psychological cause; i.e., when not confident enough to address an issue and in crisis, one may be tempted to alter the normal pattern of one's thought and speech, adopting a stutter, hissing 'c's and 's's and other means of getting people to ask "What caused this?", so that help would be forthcoming with the difficulty one wasn't confident enough to confront alone.

To be honest, everyone wants to maximise their abilities to think and talk so that they can help themselves and others as much as possible, and making it hard to communicate just aggravates the situation.

If you're under stress and tempted to go off on this tangent to the real solution of the problem, bear in mind that most people don't have Judy Moody's understanding of this cause of speech defects and won't ask "Why?", and you'll be lumbered.

51. Flowers, Music and Love

Louisa Mew worked with Jack Michael Mackintosh and Laurence O'Lansa at a florist's shop. What was unusual about this flower business was the fact that the male employees outnumbered the female, the above were the 'team' managed by the last mentioned.

Lou was approachable and caring, indeed this fact outweighed the deficiencies of procrastination, being easily distracted and casting doubt on everything, which were faults also possessed by her. Nevertheless, she is valued by her colleagues and regular customers alike.
She and Larry in turn hold J Mick Mac. in high esteem as he has been in the trade since leaving school, as were his parents before him. Give Mick a petal of any flower and he will identify it, giving it's Latin as well as its common name. Mick Mac. is a joker, but can keep a straight face too, so Larry cannot tell whether or not Mick is being serious.

Larry is just a little younger than Lou, who is nearly Mick's age, 50 years old. They are single, but have had partners of the opposite sex which all came to nothing.

It seemed to Jack Mac. that Lou was increasingly caring towards Larry, who shared her passion for opera. They went to the local venues together whenever an operatic performance was produced, and, it seemed to J. M. Mac. that Larry, younger, good-looking with oodles of charm, might be an attractive proposition for Lou.

It was in Mac's nature that he said what was on his mind, so he mentioned in an everyday conversation he had with Lou that he thought they made a nice couple. Lou was aghast and said "I might go to the opera with him, but I would never marry O'Lansa!".

52. Little Spherical Things

I am writing in this place for the few faces that can appreciate great mini-masterpieces of literature.

Anyone who has read my previous work will be expecting me to make a profound philosophical statement in an amusing manner.

They will be disappointed, for I intend to write a piece encompassing trivia and drivel in a tedious, tendentious and boring way.

You may wonder why I am doing this, and the answer is that it will provide a tremendous challenge for me not to produce a work seemingly divinely inspired. The difficulty I face is overcoming years of mental exercise, in order to write in a seemingly brain-numbed way.

However, here I go.

Once upon a hill stood a girl still willing to fill her life with glorious moments of ecstasy (imagine the pleasures of eating an éclair, drinking champagne, and lying by a pool in L.A., with the person you find the most attractive in the world).

This girl knew Hell in the past, and was now heading for Heaven on Earth through embracing love, truth, beauty, strength, goodness, right and happiness, in a bid to overcome her historical problems.

You may ask, "Why make the effort? Why bother?" She could stay miserable all her life and deteriorate. God would probably forgive her.

I would reply that it is her duty and common sense tells her to achieve this.

Oh dear! Have I done it again?

53. Madame Jeanne Recamier

Benny and Penny Henney had three sons and one daughter who faced many choices just the same as everyone else.

Choices over what to know, believe, think, do, say, and the opposites. The eldest son, Kenny, proved an inspired guide to younger brothers Denny and Lenny and their little sister Jenny.

Kenny made the decision early in life to be as good as possible, with a belief, sustained throughout his presence on Earth, in truth being it's basis. Whatever situation he faced he ascertained the facts, and acted according to the relative merits of the different positions of what was in question.

Don't get me wrong, Kenny wasn't infallible and did err on occasion. However, with his strong conscience behind him enabling him to, with hindsight, correct the mistakes and act to positively fulfil his omissions, he kept on the straight and narrow pathway that promoted peace of mind.

If only I had been such an example much earlier in my life as some individuals I've known are.

54. Too Fast

Henry D Hendy had a huge horse that he rode, a la mode, till it stepped on a toad. "Oh woe" said Henry "your toe has tramped on an innocent being, bringing about it's expiration. What will transpire for Tarquin the toad now he's been terminated?"

Although the question was rhetorical, it raised the eyebrows of Elias, the horse, who had feelings of guilt for bringing about the demise of what had been, in its own way, a handsome male.

Elias trusted that Tarquin would be judged by the 'Creator of All' on his merits whilst alive; "This seems only fair", he surmised.

Henry, although he didn't put it into words, felt likewise, and learnt a lesson from this loss of life.

"Never again, Elias," he said to his transport, "will we go so fast that we are unable to avoid taking the temporary time remaining of a single soul, ending it's existence accidentally."

Speed, though thrilling, is responsible for killing and maiming many minions of the Almighty who should be surviving satisfactorily. Please ensure that you're so slow everyone and everything you encounter is safe and the sound and sight of an iniquitous incident is absent.

THE PREVIOUS ESSAYS OF A FORMER PARANOID SCHIZOPHRENIC

Incidentally, all the characters and events in this story are fictitious and bear no relation to anyone or anything living or dead.

55. Scream: The Registry

There he was in a bar again, surrounded by gorgeous young creatures. The bar staff were nice too.

It can be surprising to one deprived of love and care, how wonderful individuals can be, and this was reinforced when Pete met Delilah.

Delilah had a very pretty face, with long brunette hair tied back. She wore a black tee-shirt and jeans and was exuberant. Who wouldn't have joie de vivre with her attributes?

Indeed, she has so much love to give that it will take one man a lifetime to exhaust it ,and even then it shall be carried over into the next realm, where only love, wisdom and goodness are felt or experienced.

This holiday from eternal life which is spent on Earth can prove such an interesting interlude, with sin, unknown in Heaven, interfering with the inhabitants' decisions. The daily battle against temptation keeps one on one's toes while the pursuit of right and truth takes place.

To make a point should be what I do next, but I will leave it to the reader to guess what Pete and Delilah did to fulfil themselves and God's wishes.

Needless to say it made them happy.

56. Capture the Rapture

Harriett Haversham-Faversham and William Wilverley-Waverley were solicitors, working for Cavendish-Davenport Ltd. of the City of London. Harri and Willi had both taken firsts in their LLB's at Cambridge, though two years separated their scholastic achievements.

While at university they had been prominent Labour activists, and had high hopes of changing the country's status quo, with the same conviction that had afforded them the self-determination in shaping their own personal destinies to the form that they truly desired, despite being handicapped by middle-class upbringings.

They no longer found that they could support ambition, satiating financial security at the expense of their moral and spiritual beliefs, to the extent where both gave up their lucrative livings in London to represent constituencies in the Home Counties at about half the remuneration that they had previously had in the city, as Members of Parliament.

Because of, or perhaps despite, their parallel careers, they obviously found lots in common with each other, and this, combined with shared ideologies, meant that eventually they found that each couldn't keep their hands off the other.

With due decorum they romanced, while discussing delicate issues of the day, together valuing the other's views immensely as respect demands.

Their marriage ceremony, though a private affair, brought politicians of all persuasions to Marylebone Register Office. For most could see that Harri and Willi were, and would increasingly become, a force to be reckoned with.

Though no-one could have foreseen how much. Within twenty-five years, with many minor and not so minor political appointments having been held by both of them, they became the first wedded couple to hold the positions of the Premiership and Deputy Premiership simultaneously.

They brought honour to politics through behaving according to, and promoting, their utilitarian and humanitarian views. Individuals can make a difference, especially in pairs.

57. The Pig Pen : This Penny Is A Copper; The Pen is Mightier Than The Truncheon

PC Penny Penelope Penfold is employed part-time by a County Constabulary. She has been, since the birth of her son Pendragon.

Penny had wanted to be a police officer since she was a child, and continued wanting to be a copper while she was a teeny-bopper and after, until she joined the aforementioned force as a special constable as a preliminary to becoming a fully-fledged full-time officer in 2005.

Discrimination because she is a woman and black meant that she never really had a chance of promotion, and only retains her job thanks to the forbearance deeply embedded in her strength of character, despite the sexism and racism inherent in her organisation.

To counteract and compensate for her perceived weaknesses, Penny, in her early days, started training in martial arts, and obtained a black belt and much increased self-esteem prior to continuing her education, ending this only after being awarded a master's degree in law.

In association with the constabulary's own remedial action in respect of its identified faults, Penny found her way clear to being viewed with favour by the younger police hierarchy, so much so that she is now encouraged to apply and recommended for promotion.

Which is exactly what she intends to do, not too long after her next child is born in June. She puts herself and her family first, of course.

Something along the lines of what Penny did to challenge prejudice needs to be emulated by all so-called minority members, so that society is reassured that such stigma is silly, and discrimination dangerous and damaging. Nothing is won without effort, and the result of striving is a worthwhile accomplishment.

Penny would say she couldn't have achieved so much without the support of her husband, Martin Luther Penfold.

58. Without a Mojo

Tojo Ono-Bono faced El Torro in the spectacularly bold fashion that we are used to from him, in the central arena of the Madrid's largest bullring in May 2008.

The black bull stamped and hoofed the ground prior to charging Tojo, the first Japanese matador in Spain's distinguished history, who reacted by simply stepping aside at the last safe moment and flourishing his blood-red cape in the face of the aggravated, aggrieved animal.

Tojo had grown to love bullfighting as a schoolboy in Yokohama, through viewing the sport on satellite TV and practising on farmyard stock found on the outskirts of his home town, until he visited Espana as a young man, where he impressed aficionados of this glorious game of cat and mouse with his knowledge, which had been culled in addition from examining books on the subject stimulated by an overwhelming interest.

Recommended by his grasp of theory, he obtained employment as an apprentice in order to glean experience from practice with bulls and real-life observation. Within five years, Señor Ono-Bono emerged from his training as a qualified bullfighter with a bright career outlook.

Years later, after reaching the pinnacle of positive prospects, he renounced his previous behaviour in which he'd gloried in gore, and now campaigns against blood sports. He has also adopted veganism for his diet.

This was after several setbacks in his private life gave rise to a response in the development of his personal philosophy, which prevents the pursuit of the deaths of living things.

However, he didn't become bitter about the damage he'd done throughout his time in the bullring and restaurants, because he embraced forgiveness for his own and others' transgressions.

It takes guts to admit mistakes and replace the thinking behind them, but this needs to be done before it's too late.

59. Human Divinity

Xavier Javier's behaviour was exemplary. From morning till night, Monday to Sunday, every week of each year of his life, he acted according to norms and values appropriate to the holy man he became, which is indeed what he achieved from his allotted timespan on this planet.

Not riches, fame, influence, power, good looks, only the wholesome moral integrity that was the basis of a daily performance that illustrated compassion, empathy, love, and, some would say, divinity.

However, he was humble in the realisation that everyone has a soul, and his is only one of the totality of all the souls that there will have been, which is what we may refer to as God.

He knew that our souls can be correctly interpreted by our thoughts to ascertain our wishes, which we shall subsequently aim to attain the satisfaction of.

It was his conviction that, as we believe all our thoughts, if we think something wrong, it will affect our behaviour detrimentally, leading to the inappropriateness we call evil.

Understanding this led him to an absence of condemnation whilst acknowledging the human frailty that prevents us correcting our errors.

These weaknesses can be minimised by having confidence and faith in the limitless ability of ourselves and others to right mistakes, given time, and become genuine people living in reality.

60. Mass Destruction

I rebuke Luke Duke for saying he'd nuke Baghdad if the car bombings continued, after pulling out US troops. Great violence is not the answer to smaller violence, although it may make the perpetrators of the latter perish. But, as has been proved, there will always be fools waiting to follow in their footsteps, while what about the innocent?

I agree with Pablo Pavlova, who states that the sooner Iraq is self-governing and foreign meddling in its internal affairs ceases the better.

Yet again an entire culture was based upon the murderous inclinations of one individual, and it was maybe necessary to excise the weaknesses of his regime and replace it with the strength of supported democratic institutions with the good of the majority at it's heart, and protection for minorities.

Easy to say. Meanwhile, people willing to risk their own and others' lives for their political masters and a regular income are being killed, as well as the uninvolved. What a bloody mess!

But nothing is perfect; life may be unfair. If only everyone refused to hurt themselves and/or others and insisted on being kind to all, what a difference it would make. Isn't this our personal responsibility?

61. Zeitgeist

Zoltan and Zola Zorab and her brother Zachary Zager weren't just a bit bizarre, but very strange indeed.

It must be said that Zola and Zachary came from somewhat weird stock, which seems to account for her choice of partner, Zoltan, and certainly her previous fiancé Zebedee. If ever you've come across odd entities then you'll know what I mean about these nonentities.

It wasn't as if they presented plausibly. Initial acquaintance produced questions in one's mind about the causes of their unusual appearance and dysfunctional behaviour, which go further than mere choice into coercion.

Surely very few people would agree to be like this unless their responsibility had been drastically diminished by emotional pressure and cruelty in their formative years, and/or maybe good intentions, leading to what must be purgatory on Earth for them? There is something artificial and affected about their attitudes, influenced by insincerity and lack of genuineness, pretence, perhaps.

Although maintaining a reasonably good standard of living primarily through greed and meanness, their quality of life cannot provide much satisfaction as they appreciate little.

THE PREVIOUS ESSAYS OF A FORMER PARANOID SCHIZOPHRENIC

Life can be long, and if the time is not used constructively the resulting neglect and deterioration can be disastrous. Motivation to restore one's equilibrium should be maximised, but it has to come from oneself, from within, (though encouragement can be of especial significance).

Only believing the truth of one's experience will lead to realising reality and real relationships in a fruitful and worthwhile way in this wonderful world.

62. Struth, is that the Truth?

Brian Briar-Cryer and Diane Dyer-Fryer seemed, from the outset, destined to share their fates.
They met during higher education, when B.B-C pointed out a dire liar to D.D-F, and tried to direct her away from the mire that dishonesty creates by giving her the advice, which she embraced, derived from a wisdom possessed by those of older years, that led her to self-examination through introspection before coming to the conclusion that, in order to be truly happy, it is necessary to overcome one's fears for the future by correcting the mistakes one has made in the past.

She came to understand that to be a real, genuine, self-fulfilling person one needs to have interpreted all past and present experience rightly, so that one acts appropriately spontaneously according to the circumstances.

Bri and Di did marry, and Bri sired and Di carried a baby boy, Guy, who absorbed these mores and values throughout his young life, recognising their validity and agreeing with them, leading to the stable childhood from which achievement flourishes easily.

Do all good people agree with the humble Briar-Cryer-Dyer-Fryers, I ask you?

63. Choice

Nolan Bolan-Dolan was the type of chap that you'd like your daughter to marry. Not that you'd guess it from his background, but it was obvious from his present demeanour and behaviour that he is the full ticket and a very wholesome individual. The real question is "Have I raised my daughter well enough to be attractive to the likes of Nolan?"

If I know you then the answer is that you did your best pragmatically to ensure your daughter's happiness, with this guiding the behaviour that would achieve her fulfilment.

So was your best good enough? Maisy Daisy, as you named her, is not lazy but self-motivated, and determined to attempt personally the implementation of her ideals, with love and goodness forming the bases of them.

She is bright, good-looking, nice and caring, with respect because of the uniqueness of each individual. She always made an effort to make the most of her attributes, spiritual, mental and physical, and developed into a most pleasant person with whom it is a pleasure to spend time.
Her personality and character leave nothing to be desired. She has it all.

However, she isn't convinced of her own perfection, as she struggles to improve and become a better example to others. I guess she acknowledges faults within herself that aren't obvious to others.

I trust Maisy Daisy's judgement in her choice of friends and lovers, and if she does ever meet Nolan there will be fireworks of fun evident with a lifetime of fantastic, fabulous, soul-enriching feasts of merriment and good works. Whilst even if she doesn't, she'll fall in love with another appropriate peer with a similar result.

64. Rust's Remedy

I shared a dormitory in Cheltenham with a degenerate reprobate called Magnusson Minor. His brother Magnusson Major was in the sixth form while we were fourth formers.

Despite his inadequacies there was something about Magnusson Minor that one couldn't help liking. Perhaps it was this that persuaded a master, Reuben Rust, to take an interest in him, or maybe R.R. believed it was part of his calling to save young Thor's soul from it's probable fate.
Whatever it's cause, Reuben's intervention was the turning point that enabled Thor to stop straying from the straight and narrow. It was the catalyst of tremendous development, and consisted purely of philosophy appertaining practically to why we are here.

Reuben had ideas that made the provision of pursuit of produced ideals imperative. These ideas, simply stated, were that each individual has a soul, with it's to desires to achieve, at his very core. Around this are his emotions, and possibly fear. On the next level are his thoughts which, if truthful, use all the information his senses provide, to guide his body's behaviour and interaction with the world to fulfil his soul's wishes.

As can be deduced, emotions and fear may prevent truthful thoughts, as might ignorance, which would result in behaviour deviating from the wise accomplishment of possible perfection to the detriment of all.

This possible perfection is manifested personally in happiness, which ultimately equates with possession and acknowledgement, through thought, of the truth.

Thor saw the sense in Reuben's statements, and turned over a new leaf. In future he would be known no longer as a malcontent, but rather as someone who had seen the light, taken a shine to it, and illuminated the lives of all those he came into contact with, with a beneficial ripple effect and a working life bringing benefits to beings through his beliefs in consummating the aims and ambitions he was born with.

THE PREVIOUS ESSAYS OF A FORMER PARANOID SCHIZOPHRENIC

65. Somewhat of a Success

Troy, Brett, Duwayne and Leroy were performers in the tribute band 'Uriah Cheap', which celebrated the work of the artistes whose heyday was before any of the aforementioned were born.

They played gigs in and around their base of Portsmouth, with occasional trips further afield.
This was a manufactured band, brought together by a big fan of the original group who rejoiced in the name of Napoleon Wellington. His Parisian mother, Wilhelmina, had always revered the notorious Emperor of the French and had only married Adolph Wellington, despite reservations about his surname, after finding herself pregnant with his child.

'The Cheapsters', as they informally called themselves, all had day jobs, but enjoyed the band socially and financially, as they were handsomely rewarded for their musical efforts by both groupies and their management. Not only that, but performing itself gave them a kick, despite having to 'dress up' in sixties gear and grow their hair extremely long. They looked and sounded the business, really quite authentic.

This was exactly what Napoleon had intended from the outset, and he was very pleased with his protégées' presentation in all its aspects, and their progress from being purely a pub band to playing larger venues and beginning to break into the festival circuit.

Although the band members appreciated the attention they were accorded, after several years of only playing what the original band had written, they started to feel restricted, so then began writing songs of their own in that style and developing the genre.

This move proved terrifically successful and, after landing a record deal, they went on to sell hundreds of thousands of a début CD of their own material. Their subsequent releases eclipsed this sales figure and the boys, by now full-time professionals, found themselves top of the bill nationwide. It only struck them how far they had come when they headlined a tour supported by the original 'Uriah Heep'.

THE PREVIOUS ESSAYS OF A FORMER PARANOID SCHIZOPHRENIC

66. Siamese Kat

Barrington Bennington-Billington visited Billingsgate often, in a quest for fresh fish. One of his great joys was masticating trout, rainbow preferably.

On several trips to this market he remarked to himself on the prettiness of a particular assistant of the noted fishmonger, Pennington-Parker, whose name appeared to be Kat.

This young lady was quite polite, and seemed very fetching in her little white cap, white coat and blue and white vertically striped apron.

After pondering upon proposing a proposition to this female, Barry, as he called himself, planned purposefully to promote agreement with Kat to proceed to a picture-house, in due course.

So accordingly, seemingly spontaneously, he approached the desirable assistant several weeks running for her assistance in his purchases, engaging in light humour and repartee, to find the girl responding and even evincing interest in his appearance at her place of employment.

Seeming to smell success in his grasp, Barry wished to find out more about this oriental temptress, and questioned her about her origins and plans.

It turned out that Kat's parents were from Persia, where her father had been a carpet exporter who had enjoyed his job very much until the magic wore off and his business crashed. Apparently he left Siam one step ahead of his creditors to live in the land of the fee, England, where all except nature costs money.

Hence Kat selling fish, her mother breeding cats and her father reduced to painting the dots on dominoes in a games manufacturing company. It was Kat's dream to restore the family fortunes by means fair or foul (or fish).

Barry expressed empathy as he pieced together her story in its entirety, but wondered if he should still woo a woman who believed that the end justifies the means. Surely, he thought, by employing only good methods the appropriate reward would follow. Whereas Kat was willing to do wrong for a right result. She came to lose Barrington.

67. Involvement

Mister Maldwyn Welsh-Dragon hailed from Cardiff, and only remained living in Hythe because he had fallen in love with Elizabeth English-Rose, a barmaid employed by Redmond Lyon who himself had strong feelings for the manageress of a pub near his own, in that locality, who was called Naomi White-Swann. Maldwyn was a keen darts player, and represented Red Lyon's pub, 'The Pig and Whistle' against White-Swann's hostelry 'The Peg and Parrot', when they had a fixture in the autumn of 2008.

Harold Fitzherbert-Farquarson was the captain of Maldwyn's team, while the opposition was led by Percy Byatt-Pyatt. These two had almost a century of playing darts between them, and although these days they rely on spectacles for perfect performance vision, they are very skilful individuals who have a fund of amusing stores, anecdotes and jokes that they have a fondness for relating in their own locals. Also in Harold and Maldwyn's team were Brian Boreham-Boram and Paul Pheasant-Partridge. While Percy had a courting couple, Shane-Wayne Payne-Caine and Kayleigh Hayley Bailey, as well as Connor-Donald O'Connell-O'Donnell, on his side.

Despite it being unusual having a woman player in men's darts this was accepted here by all, as Kayleigh is so sociable and competent, 'one of the lads' you could say; besides, Shane-Wayne was besotted by her, and they were inseparable.

Both teams had their supporters with Elizabeth and Red leading one group and Naomi leading the other in this good-natured affair at The Peg and Parrot, although it was a crucial match for each of them.

First one team would lead, then this would alternate, and towards the end they were neck and neck, but most weren't disappointed by the final result as friendships had been cultivated and forged throughout the excitement.

Mr England-Ireland, the supposedly impartial umpire, voiced the belief of most present that it isn't the winning that counts but the taking part. Though this isn't always the case when it comes to winning hearts and minds in the romantic scheme of things maybe?

68. Shamrock

Dr Huntley Lunt-Punt was the country gentleman and dentist who extracted a decaying tooth from the mouth of Ruth Booth, who subsequently told the truth to Craig Haig about the plague.
Ruth was a school history teacher, and Craig one of her pupils. His step-father was the well-known Formula One racing driver, Max Lomax, who also employed Dr Lunt-Punt in his professional capacity, as did his wife Gloria Lomax.

Dr Keith Heath looked after the teeth of Huntley, working in the same practice, and was an acquaintance of Max and Glo and an avid motor sport fan.

Realising that the Irish Grand Prix was due soon, Keith asked Huntley to procure tickets for the event from the patient Max Lomax, who had an appointment for a check-up later that week.
Lunt-Punt greeted Max for his examination, and extracted a promise from him to provide two track-side passes for the race, near the pit stop, for the enthusiastic interested Heath.

Keith, also keen on bright women, and being a single man, had taken the liberty of asking Ms Booth for her phone number after Huntley had taken her tooth out and Ruth, having always fancied him, had provided it.

So now Keith rang Ruth with the offer of a weekend in Eire, as his guest, to view the biggest race in Irish history, which Max would be taking part in.

Ruth asked for certain assurances and time to consider her position, which Keith agreed to. At school the next day she mentioned to Craig that she might be going with a male friend to see his step-father in action on the Emerald Isle.

Craig told his mum that evening, and Glo Lomax suggested she chaperone Ruth as she'd be glad of the company.

Ruth called Keith and assented to go with him to Erin, subject to his acceptance of this proviso. He was delighted with this opportunity to get to know Ruth and renew his acquaintance with Gloria.

This story is so plausible I almost believe it myself, and I know I just started off with five names and went with what they evoked and rhymed with.

69. Ridiculous

Ludo Cross was my preposterous boss, usually posturing and posing, seeming to consider the pros and cons of important delicate matters when his major influence was only what was in it for him, and how the ramifications of his decisions would reflect upon him and his position.

As you can guess I never liked the man, but had to tolerate him until the day he finally convinced an alternative department of his fitness for employment with them, which was their mistake.

The only reason we were employed was to provide a service to clients, but Ludo almost solely concentrated upon pleasing those in higher posts than himself, while 'lording it' over his staff and avoiding clients wherever possible.

His need for attention was such that the staff were preoccupied with him a lot of the time instead of doing their jobs. He discussed weighty choices he had to make, such as which vehicle and caravan he should purchase, insisting they read his brochures.

When a colleague was attacked by a client in his presence he ran away and locked himself in the office. This chap was also a bully, who took advantage of his superior position to behave rudely, insultingly and dictatorially to his workers.

Of course there is something wrong with the man. It is as if he was challenged a lot, much earlier in his life, and weakly failed to respond appropriately, gradually becoming disillusioned with himself and therefore others and life, though he is anxious to appear normal, marrying and having a daughter.

One may question the judgement of his wife in choosing him to wed, but I suppose she has her own issues. Let us hope the daughter is stronger than the parents, and that her nature won't be altered by any of their perverse 'nurturing'.

70. The Story of a Scrounger

Julie Dooley loved Ray Day truly, but treated him coolly if he became unruly, as on his 18th birthday when, newly experiencing the intake of immense amounts of liquor, he got drunk.

Ray's sister, Kay Jay, was Julie's best friend throughout secondary school and beyond that time, but Ray only had interest in Julie from when he reached 16 years of age until the age of 22 when he divorced her after fathering two children by her.

Fay and May Day and their mother Julie Day, nee Dooley, experienced a life on the breadline as they were on Social Security, living in a council flat paid for by Housing Benefit. Luckily, Kay Jay, a bright, ambitious woman, went to university and, subsequently employed in business as an accountant, financed 'treats' for the kids while her brother's contribution went to the Child Support Agency. He was ill-able to afford this, as he continued fathering children until his vasectomy brought an end to this productive philandering, three children later, each by different mothers.

He soon found that the CSA expected so much money from him that he was better off on Sickness Benefit, working 'on the side'. His irresponsibility went back a long way, and had resulted in physical damage to his body through motorcycle accident injuries. He used these as a reason for being unable to work.

Some would say Ray 'lived the life of Riley', but he did have physical health problems, emotional difficulties that led to it being impossible for him to sustain relationships, poor self-esteem and, latterly, guilt, for not maintaining his several children in a satisfactory manner.

I wouldn't swap places with him; neither, I suspect, would those who criticise him for 'swinging the lead'. We only want him to do his best which, given his issues, he probably is, despite a poor quality of life and standard of living. Obviously we don't know the complete historical circumstances, if we did perhaps we could be a bit more understanding.

71. See More

There once was a very perceptive person called Seymour C. Moore, who incidentally saw more and perceived plenty through having passed important information, pure and unadulterated, from his senses to his soul and vice-versa.

His behaviour, deriving as it did from true observations correctly interpreted, both from within and without, back and forth, led to the achievement of wise accomplishments in accord with the holy love upon which all life is based, which he acknowledged, notably in relationships, especially with his attained family, consisting as it did of a wife and the son and daughter that their sexual love caused to be manifested. But being a sage didn't lead to the denial of the lighter things like laughter and humour which, when harnessed, lead to happiness, assisting the pursuit of serious conclusions concerning caring and carrying this out. Indeed, aren't the ultimate aims of all of us to be unhurt, unharmed, healed and healthy, experiencing the joy of Heaven now, on Earth, and later, in eternity?

In order to complete these aims it is necessary to review experience through hindsight, and truthfully solve the issues that, at the moment, pervert our perceptions with preconceptions.
You cannot be stopped from doing this except by your own weakness – preoccupying yourself with

comparative trivia one way or another. Will is all that's necessary. Listen, the reward is wonderfully worthwhile.

72. Permanent Parting is Such Sweet Sorrow

We did bury merry Mrs Ruby Bury-Berry in Bury St Edmunds, St Edmund's Church churchyard, after wet beriberi caused her heart to fail. An endeavour was made to prevent this, but to no avail.

Dr Dale Lale-Bale-Vale had tried to provide a diet of adequate thiamine and vitamin supplements for his mate Ruby, who he'd met on a date at the Garden Gate Restaurant, around the corner from the Golden Gate Bridge, near San Francisco, some years before. Alas too late, Gott in Himmel, for this treatment to be efficacious.

Who would have thought that this courting couple's coupling would cease and the romance end after she'd caught this terrible complaint and died before they could be married, let alone divorced in court?

Widowed Ruby Bury-Berry had eaten only polished rice and not had sufficient protein, which caused her disease, after being parted from her prospective life partner by the Atlantic Ocean when he came to work in Suffolk.

Dale sent for Ruby to join him when patient, persistent, quite probing questioning over the 'phone eventually produced disquiet in his mind over her health.

On her arrival at the English airport, seeing her symptoms, swollen limbs, the doctor was shocked and saw how some mocked her. He responded to her terrible difficulty tremendously differently, treating her delicately, mentally and physically. He loved her lots and longed for his 'cutie' to be cured, but instead catastrophe; it was curtains for Ruby.

The moral of this tale is that if you love somebody, don't leave them for a prolonged period, or you may be painfully parted permanently, forever regretfully, regrettably.

73. Acceptance

A while back, Nelly Neill-Downe knelt down on one knee when presented to her employer's guest, Manfred Rimmel-Rommel, who was descended from a prominent Junkers family, although this was really rather overdoing it.

Esther Lester-Sylvester had long been a pen pal of this particular Prussian, indeed since they were both in their teens, forty years before. She had invited him to her Holly Hill home on this occasion so that he might accompany her to an investiture, perhaps bringing, as he usually did, zing and zest to the passing of the proceedings, also because he knows how to behave in Court circles.

Esther, despite being a jester, has a serious side, devoting her able attention to the work of the International Red Cross over a sustained series of some decades, sacrificing personal pleasures for the joy of assisting others in dire need in difficult circumstances, which is why she is being rewarded by the Queen of England with an honour for this contribution acknowledged by the British Government.

However, she soon returned the insignia of her honour to Buckingham Palace, in protest at the 'hood-winking' of the public by the Premier with regard to WMD in Iraq.

Even the privileged especially can possess principles.

74. The Fight Against Filth

Dean Keane-McLean was keen on keeping things clean. He'd say, "A clean ship is a happy ship". It was as if his boat came in when things were spick and span. He'd push the boat out again after spring-cleaning, finding it not in the least demeaning, more meaningful than merry-making, longer lasting than laughing, superficially superior to smiling.

But, expending elbow grease in the conquering of grime made him happy, a cheerful chappy. It gave him a raison d'etre, each mission in the cause of cleanliness as successful as could be. He was never weary of wiping surfaces, he only wept when dirt dictated.

Disinfectant, bleach and anti-bacterial spray were his closest allies in this fight against filth, battles fought frequently. There were no tears when every room was totally tidy, neat and spotless.

He was house-proud, and hours of housework provided his pride. Presently personally I prefer alternative preoccupations in the pursuit of pleasurable periods, perhaps in the pub.

75. Hugh Mee

Messrs Hume and B. Ing were serenely, supremely, somewhat surreally satisfied with life as human beings. They found that all they needed to do to be happy was to relax, chill out, and take their time to think the truth as soon as possible without procrastination, while choosing to be good in all circumstances.

They neglected to humour the Devil, which made the Creator cheerfully disposed to ensure that their behaviour was rewarded with joy and glorious moments of eternal ecstasy in the afterlife, and an appreciation of a high quality of life beforehand.

I reckon that you are wondering what the catch is. But El Diablo is bluffing by engendering such cynicism. Life is simple and straightforward. Be good by thinking correct thoughts of our desires and experience, past and present, and do, think and say right. Strive to be fearless.

76. Everyday Awe

Alphonse Ponsonby presupposed many things, manufacturing reasons why his life should be miserable in the future, as it had always been for him.

However, experience gleaned from his peers and certain individuals who are inspirational indicated to this immature man that passing time could be a pleasure when we've taken the opportunity to plan positive pursuits producing the product of pleasing The Great Provider of Paradise, who rewards such conduct with a quality of life of a standard according to the effort and determination employed.

Acknowledging the information his senses provide, and interpreting it spontaneously, truthfully, became Al's Holy Grail, and, decades later, his achievement. Now he could modify unsatisfactory situations.

He thanks all those who guided him in this quest; marvellous, almost awe-inspiring, ordinary mortals who have just been honest.

77. J.D.

Tod Dodd believed in God, while his erstwhile friend Oscar Oswald was obviously oblivious to the idea of an extra especially exceedingly exquisite entity existing, a Creator consisting of indestructible goodness, who is forgiving of the deliberate and accidental mistakes mere mortals may make that lead to bad behaviour.

Tod was convinced that man and womankind would be judged on their merits against the positive potential that they will have had in time. He therefore decided to be as good as he could be, as it is right, thinking that this might also compensate a little for those who weren't like that or who were actually bad, while Oscar chose to be good as it is natural to be thus, in spite of the fact that some are bad. So, are you good to make up for some who are bad, or despite some being bad, or is it simply that you realise this to be your true desire?

Although I additionally accept that all will be forgiven, I realise that considering the particular circumstances of the individual, the appropriate reward will be accorded to that person on Judgement Day, so, personally, I really want to be at my most deserving then.

THE PREVIOUS ESSAYS OF A FORMER PARANOID SCHIZOPHRENIC

78. Ma Belle Amie

My beautiful friend, Belle Bellamy, had a face that rang a bell, in that if you had ever imagined a vision of a visage of loveliness then this was it.

Not only that, but her character and personality portrayed potential perfection, with charm and friendliness being their most disarming and salient features.

Indeed, she is also so humble, realising that looks are only a peripheral attraction and that her many qualities and more can be shared by all with ambition to achieve sharing an afterlife with the Almighty.

She sees that each and every individual is equal, with innocence and a belief in truth being available to all, while a life dedicated to choosing good in chaotic circumstances is the best way to go on and the only way to satisfy souls.

It wasn't until I'd read the above that I saw I'd been writing about Pauline Nolan, a special lady, who died on 14th March 1998, aged 51, from breast cancer.

She is greatly missed, and her contribution to my well-being and others cannot be over-estimated.

Belle Bellamy is Pauline Nolan.

79. Mates

Pretty Biddy Priddy met nice Bryce Rees-Rice when she was out one evening with seriously heavy Heather Heaver-Leaver. The latter was chatted up by sparkling Jules Kewell-Jewell, himself a strapping 6ft 3ins and 18 stone.

Jules and Bryce had become friends at a local football club, which they had attended regularly for training and playing purposes since the year 2006. Both being single, they socialised together, drinking and introducing themselves to women in bars and clubs.

Seeing Biddy attracted Bryce as he has good taste, and wouldn't waste an opportunity to get to know Biddy and allow her to show and demonstrate a personality illustrating a good nature, which included remonstrating over iniquities and unfairness.

Despite being overweight, Heather herself was still shapely, and possessed a charming and bright outlook, some would say scintillating, although she doesn't sin much. Jules was impressed, as she is much more than just not repressed or depressed. Indeed, he thought, "What more can I ask for? I'm on to a winner here."

So both the men did the obvious, and provided amusing and intelligent company for the women, who, in their shy, respectable ways, welcomed these opening moves towards a later seduction, while checking out that the fellows were of the wholesome character that would make them deserving of success.

Once this was established the men and women's mutual respect led to a period of romance that culminated initially in Bryce and Biddy's engagement, and latterly, to Jules and Heather living together.

Despite all life's trials and tribulations, these four individuals stayed in contact for the rest of their lives, being there for each other when needed and giving support where possible.

I think that the value of lifelong relationships, which always start off as strangers becoming friends, is inestimable.

80. Believable

Archduke Marmaduke Charmaduke presented Bill Ball-Bell with a bauble that the babble of the rabble said was a great honour.

He was recommended for this trinket by Sgt. Bill Coe, a not officious official, who had witnessed today's invested individual providing Major De'ath, the army undertaker, with several customers who were in the wrong place at the wrong time, a current theatre of war.

A million vermilion wounds inflicted upon an enemy apparently prove that one's country is in the right and doing well, but this is just the Devil's evil spreading misapprehension. The truth of the matter is that killing foreign strangers is as insane as capital punishment is for convicted murderers, and we now acknowledge that this is wrong.

Awarding medals to killers, in my opinion, lowers the prestige and makes base the currency of reward for service to society. Those who sacrifice souls should be shunned, instead of being sensationalised as something special.

81. Receive and Transmit

The extraordinary Audrey and Aubrey Auden agreed that though through thorough thought the correct conclusions could become crystallised, too many minions of the Almighty make the mistake of omitting to often offer an effort to achieve this aim, with the result that satisfactory solutions, seemingly not sought, don't materialise. Ignorance is ignoble, ingratiating the individual with the icon of evil idols.

Constant consultation and questioning can conclude quite quietly in contemplative consideration of key issues.

Aud. and Aub. Aud. now know complete knowledge of the truths their senses tell, never will disturb or distress them, while refusing to admit such truth shall and should terrify them until they find the strength to think the facts their senses feature.

82. Unusually

Freddie Fountain-Waters helped Fleur Flowers-Bloom blossom into an incredibly attractive individual through an input of love, the like of which Fleur hadn't experienced in her life before.

This romance was sustained over a number of years and led to marriage, and Freddie became so happy with his lot that he couldn't foresee disaster on the horizon.

Indeed, a Machiavellian melodrama was about to unfold as Wilbur Wedlock-Warlock persuaded naïve Fleur that she had led a sheltered life, and needed to chill out in order to be cool.

Part of this process proceeded in the form of imbibing bottles of WKD, until Fleur's so-called friend, Carrie Parry, invited Fleur to accompany her and Wilbur back to their gaff near the Jackpot Café.

Fleur, rather the worse for wear, unwisely agreed. Back at their pad, Wilbur lit up a joint and passed it around, with vodka and lemonade and Jack Daniels and Coke flowing freely.

Inebriated Fleur, anxious not to offend and unassertive, impassively, passively, puffed pensively. Presently Barry, Carrie's brother, stumbled drunkenly into the flat and took the opportunity, presented as planned, to take advantage of the innocent, innocuous wife of Freddie, who was unfortunately unavoidably detained elsewhere looking after a sick relative, now she was in no condition to say no.

These three conspirators had mixed, malicious motives for making Fleur feel distraught, including jealousy and sadistic, evil tendencies and they couldn't wait to tease timid Freddie about this debacle.

However, Freddie forgave these three fiends and Fleur, whom he considered a victim. Fleur couldn't forgive herself for many years for being so foolish and letting Freddie down.

83. Mecca

Patsy Pattingham-Passingham, Miss Australia, the outgoing Miss World, crowned Miss Italy, Sophia Spinelli-Spinetti, the next Miss World after the judges had decided that she is the most attractive woman on Earth now.

Though the reasons for their decision may be rather spurious, I do find their choice particularly pleasing, presupposing that certain assumptions I've made appertaining to her possible perfection prove probably plausibly positive.

Sophia seems sweet, harnessing humility and humanity, being incredibly incredulous over her win, her character reflecting reliable reasoning regarding reality and a personality portraying personal qualities of an enormous quantity.

Indeed, if she is as good as she is beautiful then she will be Saint Sophia, an angel, a contender for one of Heaven's thrones, if she plays her cards right.

But temptation is a funny thing, an impostor, with the evil choice masquerading as something desirable and God knows, Sophia shall be tried and tested, with opportunities to make mistakes, countless in number, on her horizon.

Patsy previously had concluded during her reign that beauty isn't a gift for life, for it to continue it must be paid for and justified through a respect for truth, love, right and goodness in deciding what to know, think, believe, do and say in response to our experiences of others, which may be personally chosen by us or otherwise inflicted, so that we grow, healing the damage that threatens to destroy us. I tend to agree with her

84. Risk

Varied various vicious village villains visited Venice very infrequently. Freaks they were, by name and nature.

There was Simon Simian, a chimpish, impish infidel who inevitably practised infidelity, in addition to finding in Hugh Mann inhumane behaviour, and that impudent prude Prudence who was being imprudent, sometimes with Simon Simian Esquire.

I could go on and mention barking Farquhar Barker and his cousin 'Nosey' Parker Harker, or Shelley with the belly like jelly, but this could be counter-productive as it might engender disinterest in the reader, perhaps it does? I've taken a chance.

If by chance you are still examining this essay, you may be wondering where it is leading. So am I.

Where shall we go with it? We have a gang of ruffians in Venice; do they sink a gondola and drown? Are they arrested? What trouble do they cause?

To be quite honest, I think this may only be of interest to the Venetian Constabulary, so I'll pass on the personal details of these individuals to them.

It may be quicker if you get on your mobile to them with this information, as I don't have one.

85. Who, Me?

Rory-Ray-Roy Lenham-Langham-Langton was resolute in seeking a solution to his present problems by resolving to solve his historic issues through correcting the mistakes he had made in the interpretation of the information certain others had provided and withheld, together with the magnification of these errors into generalisations which had upset him greatly.

Nearly five decades passed before the secrecy stopped, and Rory-Ray-Roy could face the facts and see real reality. He, metaphorically and literally, 'changed his mind' in part. Now he knows all individuals should know, think, believe and say the complete truth, this is always good, while forgiving themselves and others for making the accidental and deliberate mistakes each and every one of which lead to badness.

They need to explain their experience truthfully to themselves and others, in order to spontaneously behave appropriately and well. He can appreciate those that do this, as he does it himself now.

86. The System

Irving Irvine was concerned about his live-in girlfriend, Daisy Paisley, after she showed signs and symptoms of going crazy. She had shoved an éclair in the face of a friend, E. Clair Sinclair, after accusing her of being a sinner; "Sin by name, sin by nature," she had said.

She took Paco's tacos from another friend, Hannah Banner, saying she banned her from masticating and then digesting them, because the Mexicans had executed Emperor Maximilian in 1867, as if this explained her behaviour.

Daisy seemed to be misinterpreting the meanings of names and words, and reacting according to her incorrect conclusions. She read newspaper headlines, heard news reports and media and advertising information, believing it was all in code and meant for her personally, being about her life and thoughts.

Irving contacted Daisy's General Practitioner, Dr Henrik Kendrick, and explained his misgivings, after Daisy refused to make an appointment to see the doctor herself. The G.P. contacted the Community Mental Health Team, and a visit from a Community Psychiatric Nurse was arranged. Cher Blair, the CPN, met Daisy, who had given up her job, and reported to her team that she suspected Daisy was psychotic, suffering from paranoia.

THE PREVIOUS ESSAYS OF A FORMER PARANOID SCHIZOPHRENIC

Dr Brain-Strain of the CMHT, a consultant psychiatrist, then visited with Cher Blair, but Daisy was evasive, saying that Cher Blair was an impostor as her name rhymed with E. Clair Sinclair's, and that this was a ruse of E. Clair's to get her own back. Daisy, having no insight into her illness, refused to go to the local psychiatric hospital as a voluntary patient, and, for reasons of her own, then stopped eating for weeks. It was only when her physical health was at risk that Dr Kendrick and Dr Brain-Strain could commit Daisy compulsorily to the psychiatric unit under a section of the Mental Health Act with the agreement of a social worker, Reid Bede.

Daisy remained at the hospital until her condition was stabilised with medication and her psychosis and paranoia minimised. However, no effort was made to discover the causes of her illness; she is expected to take medication for the rest of her life, and she hasn't been encouraged to examine her history to correct any mistakes or wrong assumptions she had previously made in life. Isn't this perhaps a sin of omission by the authorities?

87. Mind-Altering Substances

In psychedelic Philadelphia, philosophical Phillipa Penn, of the University of Pennsylvania, spotted a kaleidoscopic rainbow over the world's largest freshwater port.

She had been partying with earnest Ernest Erlinger-Singer, the vocalist in the band The Benjamin Franklin Swingers, of the Franklin Institute.

I can certainly surmise with some certainty that this popular pair had probably previously popped some pills, for they didn't smoke, and there was no rainbow there in the sky at 3.00am this early morning. It hadn't even been raining.

Ernie had been singing with his Swingers, backed by the Philadelphia Symphony Orchestra, at a charity function in Pennsylvania's biggest concert venue, while Phillipa viewed from the wings of the stage.

The post-performance party attracted many profligates, and unfortunately unprescribed medication was in proliferation. Phillipa wasn't alone in suffering the symptoms of drug abuse, for her partner Ernie entertained tolerance for experimentation with illegal substances, and early signs of psychosis could be detected in Ernie's psyche by those in possession of psychiatric knowledge. However, help wasn't forthcoming at this point.

Ernie's lack of insight eventually led to insanity or, to coin a phrase, mental health difficulties, after serious serial sessions with several illicit substances, especially speed, caused him these ill-effects.

Phillipa, shocked by Mr. Erlinger-Singer's deterioration, and, luckily, undamaged by her own chemical experiences, vowed to abstain from their use totally, and went on to advocate abstinence for all, extending to and including alcohol.

Ernest Erlinger-Singer struggled with mental health difficulties for the rest of his life, relying on prescribed drugs for the alleviation of their symptoms.

Miss Penn stopped mixing with men who might lead her astray, and found fundamental fulfilment in reaching her potential for positive behaviour after theorising and constructing the personal philosophy that led to her self-actualisation, i.e., achievement of her innate desires, including procreation, but not with the likes of Ernest though.

88. Grants

Pandora Wilde-Swanne is a beautiful exotic dancer in the club, BCL's, owned jointly by Brad Chad Ladd and Brett Chet Lett. To be specific, she is a lap-dancer, and was introduced to this work by an equally attractive young French female friend of hers called Gigi Fifi Pompadou-Pompadour, who is currently studying, like Pandora, at the University of Southampton. However, Pandora is reading French, while Gigi is reading English. They converse, quite obscurely, in the language that their other company doesn't understand, ensuring privacy, but which I found really rather disconcerting initially, one night at BCL's, when I employed both to dance simultaneously for me.

Although the girls seemed to be beyond my reach, metaphorically speaking, I expressed an interest in them to Jim Gem, the head bouncer, who I've known for several years since becoming a club habitué, and he provided the details noted above. As is usual with me, I wished to forge a relationship with these two dancing girls, who had only been working in the club for nearly a month. Unfortunately I had got off to a bad start, by interjecting en Francais in their French conversation, which they'd assumed I didn't understand. They were shocked and worried that they might have said something which I found offensive, and were anxious to assure me of their goodwill, albeit in a professional capacity.

THE PREVIOUS ESSAYS OF A FORMER PARANOID SCHIZOPHRENIC

Gigi and Pandora worked at the club part-time throughout their courses of study, and I got to know them sufficiently well to become somewhat of a confidante. Enough to know that Brad and Brett, the club proprietors, who are old enough to be the girls' fathers, used their positions to obtain sexual favours from the two dancers, who felt obliged to please these men who provided them with an opportunity to earn the funds to continue their studies.

How desperate these students must have been for an income to allow the two men to take advantage of them. One can understand people 'dropping-out' of university because of financial pressures, if they feel forced to forfeit their innocence in order to forego academic failure and to ensure scholastic success.

89. Opinion Too

Deacon Parsons, Father Priest, Reverend Vicars, and Bishop Canon had one thing in common, they all believed in fantasy.

They had faith in the veracity of the contents of a book to such an extent that they based decisions and even their lives upon it.

They would quote from this book, convinced it told the story of 'The Son of God'. This was handy, as it absolved them from responsibility for their own lives and independent introspection and soul-searching. They had long since ceased to please themselves...self-actualise, and instead fulfilled conditions of worth... pleased others at their own expense.

One can obviously learn from novels, especially when they've been written to illustrate moral points, but surely passing these inventions off as fact is dangerous?

This book was based in obscure times, and about a hero who, like Superman, had miraculous powers. Calling this chap 'The Son of God' is rather pushing it, certainly insulting the Almighty.
These men were employed in religious businesses, churches, which exploit gullible and weak persons with no personal sense of direction, appealing to the goodness in their nature.

THE PREVIOUS ESSAYS OF A FORMER PARANOID SCHIZOPHRENIC

The spirit within us all, that should be nurtured with truth, is undermined by them with fictions in a concerted attempt to obtain and maintain authority over their victims, while receiving financial support from the latter and influence in society.

The 'faithful' are promised eternal life in return for believing lies, and it is only after they are dead that they discover that they were taken for a ride.

I contend it is too late then, and that the religious also need to be aware now.

90. Well Hung

Edgar-Allan Coe-Lowe-Poe recently wrote a tome, illustrated by Claude-Edward Monet-Manet, that told about how a treacherous dog called Lord Orr-Hoare, of the blessed, beloved House of Lourdes, was partially responsible for the deaths of many patriots, including Padraig 'Paddy' Padwick, Abdul Abdullah, Blaise Blaze and Iris H Irish, through the artificial dissemination of misinformation, attempting the collective deception of the inhabitants of the nook-shotten Isle of Blighty during the dull, dark, dank nights of the early 1940's.

E-A C-L-P contended that Orr-Hoare's intense irritability indicated inaccurate or insufficient introspection, but I'd argue that it was the immature response to his English ex-girlfriend, Saffron Rose, that accounted for this. His memories of her mammaries led to his ingratitude for her attitude. He had a purely puerile personality, portraying poor psychological functioning and adjustment.

The aforementioned author ascertained an apparent altitude of attitude from O-H towards the Allies, far beneath that warranted. This mistaken judgement of many may have made this man mad, surely he must have had diminished responsibility and integrity to have propagated propaganda improperly towards the peace-loving population of this sceptred isle?

THE PREVIOUS ESSAYS OF A FORMER PARANOID SCHIZOPHRENIC

Certainly, at the cessation of hostilities, public hatred for Orr-Hoare demanded that he be hanged. And so it came to pass.

Mr Coe-Lowe-Poe's book is edifying and educative and to be recommended, like this one, hopefully.

91. Three Wise Men

Methodical introspection can be metaphysically retrospective in metaphorically bringing the past to the present, inciting insight into it. At least that's what my counsellor, Councillor Count Sellers, said. I'm not sure I understand, but I think what he meant is that correspondingly consecutive memories of mistakes can be chronologically catalogued into categories, enabling consideration, so that they can be corrected currently, making the present more pleasant.

His colleague, Alderman Alderton-Alderson, also a wise one, wondered out loud if faith in fantasy fed and fuelled feeble-mindedness, forcing the fellow or female in question to act ineffectively or evilly. All I know is that the acknowledgement and realisation of reality really results in catharsis and healing, making one functionally positive.

The High Sheriff, Hugh Sharif, contended that there will be divisions within one until decisions are reached by one regarding right and wrong, resulting in resolutions to resolve the inner conflict of good versus bad, truth against untruth, strength and weakness, correct cognition and emotion.

I agree with what I believe these three men mean.

92. Recovery

Idi Otis Otway was a shot-away idiot, fathered by an African dictator and borne by a cult-comedian's sister Olive, in Ottawa. Olive married a different comedian and ornithologist called Will Oddie, and the boy became Idi O. Oddie.

Being optimistic, Idi hoped that through reflection and study he might develop wisdom and become a complete individual with an earnest and profound side to his personality, such as he had witnessed in his teachers at school.

So, with determination, he persevered in self-examination of his history and issues, and through this introspection achieved peace of mind and cognitive ability.

You see, Idi, like everyone else, wanted to use his life to make a major contribution to humanity and sensed this, despite his degeneration into the stupidity of his teenage years, it helping to motivate him in his recovery and growth.

Idi took control of his life and shaped his destiny by strengthening his character, with the certainty of correctly considering what his personal preferences in choices were, positively examining the conclusions and fears that ignorance had initiated in the light of knowledge, and replacing these with the happiness and confidence that the truth brings.

If this information isn't apparent, it is incumbent upon one to question those directly involved and to check public records, if necessary, to obtain it. That way leads to success.

A fruitless, futile future of failure is the only alternative that can possibly be featured.

93. Music

The day Simon Ryman-Wyman, Nathaniel-Daniel Hahn-Cahn and Corey-Carey Carragher-Gallagher got together to write songs is a date celebrated by their domestic and foreign legion of fans, who recognise that lyrics of love and its associated aspects are most relevant to their lives, and who also find the melodies pleasing too. For existence is caused by pleasure in love and goodness, while truth promotes this. Music, being the food of love, combined with articulations about l'amour, gives countless creatures comfort.

Correct choices and decent decisions deriving from truthful thought regarding right and wrong result in good behaviour and genuine relationships, with individuals striving strongly and successfully to sustain effort to achieve a positive outcome from every situation.

Fun, following on from publicising publicly in song how ideals may be implemented, with simple stories illustrating this together with tunes, is innocent and cannot be overrated, for they are based upon love.

Simon, Nat and Corey are disciples of God, maybe not without sin, but nevertheless guiding each of us and youth in truth, which should be the primary purpose and priority of us all.

94. No Surprise

Divine D. Vine-Devine deduced he observed a sign that Riley O'Reilly-Reilly's daughter, Kylie, had designs on him. For she spoke highly of him, to him and Riley, who imparted this information to D. Vine-Devine Senior, his golfing partner, who told his son.

Consequently, confident of the consequences of questioning Kylie about her availability, he considered chatting her up as his chosen course of action and concluded he should, so he did. God forbid anything untoward occurring in this process, Kylie responded reasonably rapidly, replying that she really had rather restricted prior engagements and a wealth of windows in her future social calendar. This being the case, V.-D. Junior, experienced encouragement in his endeavour to enlist Kylie as his prospective partner in personal pursuits and, emboldened, put it to her that they planned passing time together. Agreement was forthcoming from this nubile young beauty to her new beau, and an arrangement was made to attend the local art gallery as a matter of urgency whilst a particular exhibition was in progress.

Visiting this art show was peculiarly pleasing for Kylie as her preconceptions were dispelled, and she experienced pleasure and positive emotion from the displays of work, as well as with D. V.-D.'s company.

THE PREVIOUS ESSAYS OF A FORMER PARANOID SCHIZOPHRENIC

Having both obtained delight from sharing each other's time, they resolved to repeat the occurrence regularly, and always achieved mutual satisfaction from the effort expended and involved.

Although everything seemed so successful, I have to report that shortly afterwards Kylie felt obliged to tell V.-D. she might have given him the sexually transmitted disease that her previous boyfriend had just informed her that he had been diagnosed as having.

Neither men, nor Kylie, had taken any precautions other than her being on the contraceptive pill.

95. A Life

The remarkable Martha McArthur made a remark about her recovery which illustrated to all that this was now very nearly completely completed.

For Martha had made mistakes, and the misery these caused motivated her to make correcting them a mission. Easier said than done, for emotions had entered into the equation together with the fear that ignorance and avoidance of the truth engenders. Becoming terrified of the unknown truth after thinking the worst, and assuming that the current situation would be maintained, led to despair and deterioration in the pessimistic belief that suicide would be the preferred option in the future after the present status quo had had its perceived disastrous effect upon her.

However, Martha had under-estimated her capacity for coping with suffering and her resilience. She came to display symptoms of mental distress, and personally found these so unpleasant that she resolved to bring about their end through the resolution of the fearful issues causing them.

Martha did as much as she could alone, but then had to rely on others' change of heart and turning over a new leaf to tell her the truth they had previously withheld before she could correct her early conclusions and realise that reality could be really rather worthwhile and enjoyable, even joyous.

This summary makes the process sound simple, but it was the most difficult goal to achieve, and required the greatest effort, but the reward in terms of happiness and quality of life has no equal, and is a tribute to her thousands of correct choices over the wrong alternatives that could have been made and which would have deflected her from her chosen course... that of goodness.

96. All Are Equal

When Matt White-Black met Rita Gita Golden-Child it was lust at first sight, and later, after introductions had been made and mutual interest was established, love at first bite, following the conversation during their wait that led to the start of their initial meal together.

Matt's mother Lulu is a Zulu, and his boxing father, Tiger Boy, is from Cardiff. Tiger Boy knew Shirley Bassey from home before she became famous.

Rita's mother is a Bangladeshi, while her father is from Hong Kong. 'Golden Child' is what his former Chinese name means, and what he changed it to when coming to England to work as a Whitehall mandarin in 1990.

It must be said that these inter-racial mixes had brought about attractive appearances for Matt and Rita, but it was the way their personalities and characters harnessed their looks that enabled them to recognise each other as kindred spirits after mutual observation of their initiating and responding behaviour.

It is said that we form judgements on people in the minute or two of first meeting, and find them likeable or not on these bases, and Matt and Rita's immediate regard for the other proves the correctness of that saying, as they both share similar outlooks and values.

THE PREVIOUS ESSAYS OF A FORMER PARANOID SCHIZOPHRENIC

All things being equal, they will spend a large part of their future lives together.

97. Carnivorous Slaughterers

Thanks to an Act of Parliament in 2005, Ian Idle-Bridle can no longer hound and persecute Foxy Foxley-Fox and his extended family throughout the realm's countryside. This practice, bordering on barbarism, could be cruel almost beyond belief, and the responsible politicians must be congratulated for banning it.

How long will we have to wait for all destruction of living things in the name of sport to be damned? Shooting beautiful pheasants and other birds dead and injuring fish's heads, jaws and mouths in fishing before throwing them back in the water, or killing them, should be fiercely discouraged.

Why is creature-eating accepted? It is almost managed destruction by ordinary people of other weaker species as supply and demand dictates.

There needs to be a sea change in attitude by humans on this, their earthly domain, from one of exploitation to protection.

Our humanity shouldn't be blunted and thwarted by primitive norms and values, it should be developed to acknowledge the intrinsic worth of every life, including those of pigs, cows, sheep, chickens, and other animals and unborn human babies whose lives should be sustained and nurtured.

THE PREVIOUS ESSAYS OF A FORMER PARANOID SCHIZOPHRENIC

None of these lives should be ended for the convenience of the more powerful.

I'll alter my pattern of behaviour in this regard when the majority do. As the saying goes 'None of us are perfect'.

But let us strive to be. We can get there together, given the will.

98. Optimism

Carlton Charlton was charming in an urbane, sophisticated manner to every creature he encountered, including those not human. Kindness exuded from all his pores, and consideration, deriving from his awareness of the unique value of each living thing, was extended by him to all of them. He regretted the fact that, as a boy, he had stamped on dozens of ants on the pavement outside the front garden of his home. Also, that he is a carnivore.

Claudia Clode-Croad became acquainted with Carlton at the Conservative Club and acknowledged his qualities, sharing them as she did to a large extent, and being inspired by his example to develop them even further. Miss C.-C. was one of many to admire Mr Charlton and the only one to have won his heart so far, apart from minor youthful fancies which came to naught. While he had recognised her innocence and rejecting of wrong.

Carlton and Claudia encouraged each other to fulfil their potential and be as good as they could be, doing their best, making the right choices, respecting their integrity in an altruistic manner, forgiving themselves and others their transgressions, which they saw and attempted to understand and therefore explain.

THE PREVIOUS ESSAYS OF A FORMER PARANOID SCHIZOPHRENIC

The outlook is excellent for these two, as they daily grow stronger with new truths being thought about their and others' past, present and future, with correct interpretations of their desires for these being made by them.

I hope that many more people emulate C.C. and C. C.-C. as they deserve to.

99. Vraiment

The calmer karma charmers, Milo Marmaduke and Marmaduchess Mimi, completed their immense, mammoth, monumental life's mission by making an impassioned plea passionately for compassion to be extended to those who, like themselves and Carl Isle from Carlisle, Tony Pandy from Tonypandy and Lyn D. Hurst from Hampshire, were challenged morally and ethically in a gigantic, Gargantuan manner, a multitude of times over many years.

The recurring temptation, torment and suffering experienced by these individuals during their lives was on an elephantine, enormous scale, for it consisted of continually choosing what those terrified of the truth becoming known were keeping from them.

The reflex reactions these unlucky humans responded with were of tremendous doubts that the information supplied by their senses were right and catastrophising their history, the present and future, in ignorance of certain aspects of the past being hidden by their ascribed families.

Milo and Mimi had discovered and reconciled themselves to facts previously kept from them, and acknowledged the devastating distress that not knowing these had had upon them.

Regaining and maintaining their integrity despite this terrible, totally disagreeable situation had become of paramount importance to them, so much so that a significant part of their time was dedicated to it and, after the truth had become apparent, they were able to absorb and harness this, achieving peace of mind in the process.

They were fortunate, in that their parents had eventually told them the truth, revealing the secrets, the finding-out of which had previously obsessed and habitually preoccupied them, though being too scared to ever have asked.

Those who cannot wait and choose to believe lies about the truth denied them are damaged, and degenerate into reprobates. M. and M. beg that understanding this cause of dysfunctional behaviour be considered and forgiveness be forthcoming for those failing to fulfil certain civilised criteria because of it.

100. Medics

Affection for the afflicted was the position of the physician, Dr Arnold Yarnold, and he, together with the surgeon, Mr Sturgeon, strived to save the suffering from pain and death.

They could only do so much, providing their patients with the probability of an opportunity of more time alive on the planet, allowing them to put their house in order, ready to meet their Maker at the last possible delayed moment.

But the reason these two medical men came to public attention was the treatment they provided for the celebrated Champions League footballer, Ace Lace. In a match he had incurred a serious injury that threatened his career. However, he fully recovered, after their expertise was expended upon him. Many in the nation rejoiced, and, as it was extremely newsworthy, Scoop Jupe, a sporting journalist, focussed public interest upon this couple of members of the BMA.

So positive was the publicity that this pair enjoyed brief popularity in the kingdom, and were accorded acclaim after their self-deprecating personalities became known, while self-promoting politicians used these two doctors as a vehicle by vowing to reward them with an award in the Queen's Birthday Honours List.

THE PREVIOUS ESSAYS OF A FORMER PARANOID SCHIZOPHRENIC

Dr Yarnold and Mr Sturgeon were much too noble to be drawn into this, and indicated that any influence they may have gained be used to advocate on behalf of the National Health Service.

101. Evident

Walter Wright-Wong was not dissimilar to Simla Rosheeni Rossini-Rossellini, reaching wise decisions regarding the relative priorities of matters including life and death, love and hate, right and wrong, goodness and evil, truth and untruth, sanity and madness, happiness and misery, strength and weakness, bravery and cowardice, and finally, their manifestations in beauty or negativity.

The choices of both of them coincided, with the former of each of the opposites being the preferred option, the achievement of which they struggled to maintain or attain with their energy and time.

They found that being brave in thinking the truth led to life, love, right, goodness, sanity, happiness, strength and beauty.

The realisation that on Earth we are human and fallible gave Walter and Simla understanding and tolerance towards those who mistakenly choose to think or say untruth or do wrong, misinterpreting themselves and their desire to think and say the truth and do right, resulting in the latter of each of the opposites happening.

W.-W. and R.-R. forgive those who so do and cause pain.

It should be obvious to you all by now that Walter and Simla were made for each other, and so it is

THE PREVIOUS ESSAYS OF A FORMER PARANOID SCHIZOPHRENIC

with pleasure that I report that, since meeting, a romance has started with a future of bliss evident on the horizon which they richly deserve.

102. An Aryan Angel

After she had been granted an eternal place in the celestial afterlife, this beauty delved into Heaven's archives to examine her time on Earth, with a view to ascertaining how she could have been better in her previous incarnation as a human being. The first thing she noticed was that she had taken on board the prevailing civilisation's norms and values, rather than more supreme, sublime standards. She saw that doing this was quite common amongst the inhabitants of the known world at this time, and that those who were more adept at adapting to the spiritual dimension were tremendously respected as wise sages. They were recognised for seeing beyond the immediately obvious to the marvellous, wonderful possibilities that goodness promoted and provided. These characters were few and far between, as organised religion seduced many who should have known better, God forgive them.

This particular lady realised at this point that her greatest achievement had been to bear children and guide them to do their best, avoiding wrong and achieving right, both pre-planned and spontaneously. There can be no greater gift than life, though this brings with it the obligation to enlighten the offspring with relevant truths.

Lady Lesley, this angelic nymphet, could see that she had made mistakes in her human form, but had tried to counteract them by correcting them where possible and forgiving herself for their commission, resolving to not repeat them. She forgave everyone for everything they will ever have done, thought and said which was wrong, and also for the good things they will never have done, thought and said. At least she tried, and she couldn't be stopped.

The thing with Lesley, which she came to witness from above, was that she had striven to stimulate sinners into repenting, although she wouldn't have put it this way herself.

L.L., looking back, appreciated that although she hadn't been perfect by any means, she had lived trying to support herself and others with her every effort. Which explains why the Lord rewarded her deservedly, in his divine fashion, with a transfer to Heaven after she had eventually come to shuffle off of this mortal coil.

103. Love

Dex Dixon rang Rex Rix on Shrove Tuesday, using his mobile, from the top of the Spinnaker Tower, in Portsmouth. "What was so important?", you may ask. The answer to this was that the previous Valentine's Day, Dex had proposed marriage to Rex's sister, Pixie, and she had, just this minute, responded favourably. You see, Rex had been the initial matchmaker of this so far successful liaison, and after hugs and kisses with pretty Pixie marking this auspicious moment, Dex wanted Rex to be the first to be told the super news of the happy couple's engagement.

Rex, thrilled and delighted, although not surprised at the news, proceeded to purchase, in haste, a bottle of the finest vintage Moet and Chandon champagne that Fortnum and Mason's could provide, and share it with his father, Tex, who insisted that he had known what was in the wind since January, but who was almost as excited as Rex, despite that claim.

Tex, having made a small fortune from shares in a Texas oilfield, made big plans to splash out on fulfilling the betrothed pair's wildest dreams for a significant ceremony and splendid honeymoon in the land of their choice, Mexico.

Dex, being fiercely independent, wished to personally finance a more modest affair, but good-naturedly gave in to his future father-in-law's wishes to avoid conflict, and in acknowledgement of his fiancée's desires and ambitions, because he loved her. He also realised that fathers generally like to treat their offspring to the greatest extent their wealth will allow, and he didn't want to deny the old man this pleasure.

What Dex and Pixie had in common was that, whilst not perfect, they did their best and made a great effort to be as good as they could be, given the prevailing state of affairs, throughout their lives so far, and I see no reason why this shouldn't continue after they've created circumstances of their own choosing in the future.

I'm sure you will join me in wishing them all the best of luck, and, especially, congratulations to the affianced.

www.ingramcontent.com/pod-product-compliance
Lightning Source LLC
Chambersburg PA
CBHW021159010426
R18062100001B/R180621PG41931CBX00036B/65